Life Philosophy
for a Happy and Healthy Existence

Christiane Beerlandt

•

Life Philosophy for a Happy and Healthy Existence

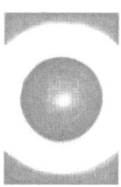

Supplement to the 1st Edition of the Book "The Key to Self-Liberation"

•

Beerlandt Publications
Lierde, Belgium

The present book contains parts of
The Key to Self-Liberation®, 2nd English edition
Written by Christiane Beerlandt®
Original title: De Sleutel tot Zelf-Bevrijding®: 1st edition 1993 – 8th, revised and expanded edition 2001 –
13th, revised and expanded edition: 2009
Copyright © 1993, 2001, 2003, 2009, 2020 by Christiane Beerlandt, Dirk Lippens (coordinating translator)
and Beerlandt Publications

Cover illustration and design by Christiane Beerlandt

ISBN: 9789075849585

Printed by InniGroup, Heule, Belgium
Bound by Brepols, Turnhout, Belgium
Legal Deposit (Wettelijk Depot): Royal Library of Belgium, Brussels
(Koninklijke Bibliotheek Albert I) D/2020/8022/4

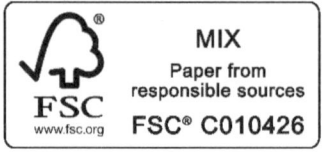

MIX
Paper from
responsible sources
FSC
www.fsc.org   FSC® C010426

The information contained in this book was meant only for educational or pedagogic purposes. The texts only
want to help and promote general well-being and were not intended for the diagnosis, the treatment, or the
healing of any disease. No part of the content of this book may be considered as a medical advice in order
to solve a certain problem. For any specific health problem, the reader has to consult a qualified health
professional. Persons with serious medical conditions have to seek professional medical care. The reader
of this book bears the full and entire responsibility for the way in which he or she uses the information contained in this book. He or she has to make use of this information in a wise, well-considered manner. No
liability whatsoever, for illness, injury, loss, or therapy, to any person, rests with the author, the translator, or
the publisher. See also the memorandum at the end of this book.

The author and the publisher decline any responsibility or liability for the content of any publication or any
website, as well as for any assertion or action by any person who pretends to base himself or herself on
Christiane Beerlandt's work. Meant are, among others, certain alternative or conventional health professionals, coaches, schools, givers of workshops, journalists. Health professionals, givers of lectures, etc. may fall
into erroneous interpretations or misunderstandings of Christiane Beerlandt's points of view or philosophy.
This can happen with the best of intentions — sometimes out of incomprehension — but sometimes also out
of ill will. Certain journalists who do not understand the heart of the matter may tear sentences from their
context which gives rise to misinterpretations. They may distort words by adjusting them to their own beliefs,
put words in the mouth of Christiane Beerlandt which she did not say, garble things — possibly causing people
to feel hurt (which is not the author's intention), cast a slur on her, insinuate things, etc.. Everything is possible
in the world in which we live. Alertness and a discerning mind are therefore required. The only sources that
render Christiane Beerlandt's vision correctly are the most recent editions of the books / texts she wrote herself.

Important Preliminary Notice

The purpose of this book is to give in-depth information about the psychological, emotional undercurrents of illness.

The author states explicitly that she is absolutely not opposed to conventional medical treatments. However, she does point out the importance of considering the underlying psychological, emotional origin of a physical disorder; she is of the opinion that this is necessary in order to achieve *fundamental healing.*

While taking a different line of approach, Christiane Beerlandt holds out a hand to medical science.

Conventional as well as alternative doctors and health professionals make use of the information from this book. It serves as a complement or as a support to the applied medical treatment.

The information from this book wants to incite the human being to self-examination when the body gives signals. It is by no means intended to point one's finger at someone else regarding their illnesses.

According to the author, there is absolutely *no question of "guilt" or punishment when one is ill;* it is merely about "failing to understand consciously" certain underlying facts. Therefore, by writing this book, the author has wanted to contribute to the human being's and humanity's becoming aware and welfare.

Christiane Beerlandt's loving devotion, her unique giftedness, and her sincere solicitude form the basis of this remarkable work.

The content of this book is intended to stimulate the human being to becoming aware; it is not meant to be used for pointing one's finger at the other with regard to his or her disease — quite the contrary. Its true purpose is to achieve greater understanding of, and deeper insight into oneself in the first place.

Communicating lovingly and respectfully, with a friend or a health professional, about the content of a certain text — without feelings of guilt or shame — has relieved much suffering and opened many eyes.

Psychosomatics and Health

For the health of a human being, it is necessary to understand the relationship between psyche and body in order to arrive at fundamental healing of mind and body.

Attention! Although the human being carries self-healing powers that are often very underestimated, most people need remedies from the outside at this evolutionary stage of humankind. Whether it's about conventional Western or other well-tried traditional forms of treatment, one can thankfully use medicine, surgery, and other treatment methods, if necessary. At the same time, one works on a solution to the psycho-emotional origins of disease and pain, while believing in oneself with rock-solid confidence — in love.

Remarks concerning this English translation

- The author wrote this book in her mother tongue, Flemish Dutch. Her style is full of images; when writing her texts, she often changed current expressions in order to convey as accurately as possible the information she "received." This makes translating her work very difficult technically. In this English version, a deliberate choice was made to remain as faithful as possible to the images in the original Flemish-Dutch text, even if this may involve some unusual phrasings, wordings or formulations in the English translation.

- About the meaning of the words "man," "he," etc., in general: Each woman, each man, could call herself or himself "man" or "he." It doesn't necessarily signify "male"; in the author's language it often means "human being," or both elements — male and female — in equality within one person. No question of discrimination.

- About the use of the word "desire": When this word is being used in the text, it always has a negative meaning: absolutely wanting to have or possess something, greediness, wanting to grab things, covetousness, etc.

A Message to the Reader

When we feel our magnificent planet Earth groan under the suffering, the violence of war, the pains, the power-game, then don't we — don't all human beings — need to take responsibility for ourselves? It is of no use to heal wounds or donate food if the underlying causes of misery are not being resolved. The world changes from within, from the inner consciousness of every human being. Illness, as well as events, are only a consequence of what happens IN the human being. If we can no longer "change" this world, then let us, each for himself, lay building blocks for a new world, where Life in its value will be understood, in Joy. There's no use screaming against, fighting against, going into the streets against. . . . True transformation begins by the human being cleansing himself of negative convictions regarding himself. Reality is only a reflection of, a result of, our unconscious and conscious expectations in life — our unconscious or conscious "steering" of energies. The future is not pre-determined, nor is life a melancholy, accidental happening about which we don't have any say. Individually and en masse, we constantly create our living world. We are in a dialogue with our planet. We don't have to wait for an Angel, a Deus ex machina, or a UFO to come and "save" the world. With the power of our Living Self, we are able to build a new house on an earth which will never be destroyed — because we wish her to be Alive.

This is possible if each of us, convinced of our loving "I AM," accepts our responsibility and no longer looks to others for the causes of illness and misery. When every human being, by himself, creates harmony in his existence, then this positive influence is a reality for all of humanity. After all, we are not separate from each other. There is more than just matter alone; energies are working more and more powerfully, including the energies which we call "emotions, awareness powers, thoughts. . . ." Let's use these energies in a Self-aware way, in growth toward health, toward healing, but also in creating a new Earth, where finally there will no longer be any suffering, pain, hunger, or death. With our feet on the ground, without floating with our heads in the clouds, let's take the helm, and become aware of the possibilities every Human Being carries inside — the possibilities of directing his existence toward something beautiful, and in so doing help lay out a feast in the nature of Mother Earth.

We need to end false determinations such as inflicting on ourselves the punishments of karma and original sin. Self-Liberation leads to the liberation of Earth and humanity. The Key that opens the gates to Joyfulness — that Key is to be found in your Self. May this book, called up from the heart "according to truth," declare its servitude as an Information-source to all good people.

Christiane
Ostend, 17 July 1993

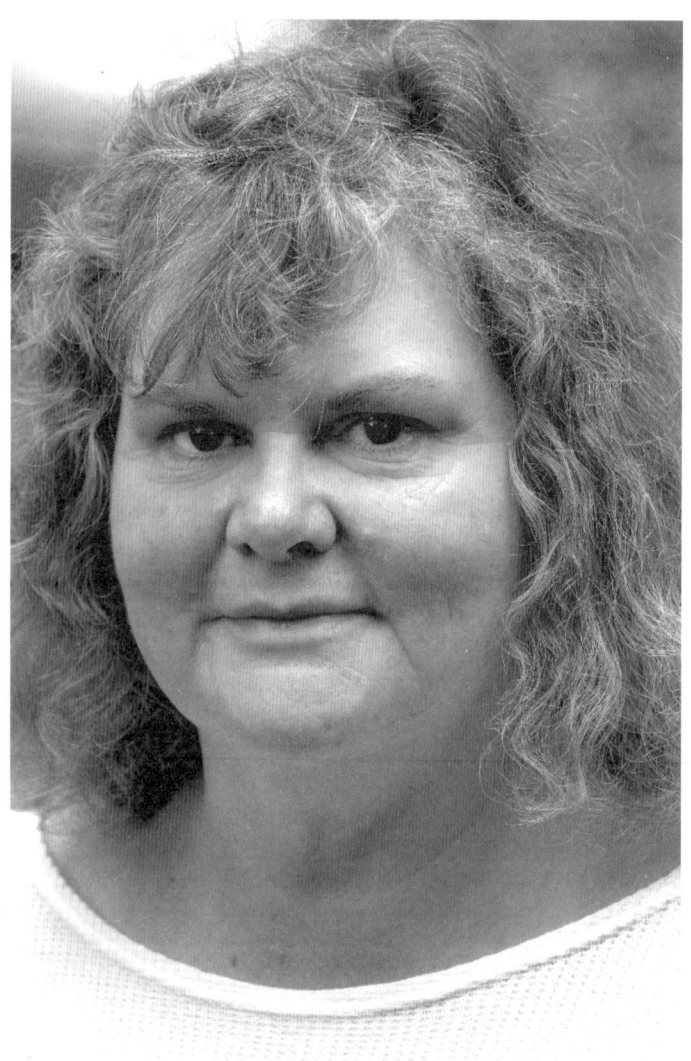

About "The Key to Self-Liberation"

It was given to me to write down *The Key to Self-Liberation* in 1992 — my first work. The information was obtained by tuning myself to the frequency of truth and listening deep inside me, via my heart and consciousness, to the deep language of life itself.

Observation and common sense are useful, but the Source of Life — via *"deeper knowing"* — reveals so much more to us: the essence, the "why" of things. No one can possess truth, not I, not you. But we can tune in to the frequency of truth, living and listening "according to truth" / in honesty. In this manner, the chapters of this book have been written. The content has nothing to do with scientific observation, but neither with channeling or guides. Don't try to pigeon-hole this book. You won't succeed. Searching people, with a "heart" and an "open mind," whether they call themselves "conservative" or "alternative," will feel at home in these chapters, which are meant to be their friends.

Even if it's not possible yet, I am convinced that "science" will come to the same conclusions as the information in this book, be it via other routes. But the "equipment" to measure psyche, emotions, and energetic happenings / evolution — the relationship between the inner self and the physical body (illness-health) — does not yet exist or is still inadequate.

For the countless "conventional" and "alternative" doctors, health professionals, and laypeople who already have worked with the information of this book for years and made contact with me, there doesn't need to be any further "proof." . . . "It simply works like that in daily life." It makes me extremely happy: how the human being can liberate and heal himself, as long as he gains "insight" and suits the action to the word — with or without remedies from the outside. **How the seeds of illness are sown**, and how we can bring about fundamental healing via Insight and Application.

Our "spiritual energy" influences the body / "matter" and not the reverse. Everything is being directed and driven from within. When we better understand these processes, we can, as conscious people, bring about change in ourselves. It has often been seen how, in certain people, acquiring "insight," or something being "triggered off" in one's mind regarding the true cause of one's illness — was enough to bring about sudden recovery. Mostly, however, we are involved with a growth process whereby the (sick) body reacts in a growing way to the changes one brings about in oneself: changes on the psychological and emotional levels, changes in one's convictions. The body reacts to those positive, necessary changes . . . and healing becomes a possibility.

I am not at all against medicine or other remedies from the outside. On the contrary, it can be good for many people to use them in a certain phase (even though many heal themselves without them). *Therefore, don't worry about using medicine or treatment methods if you feel this is best for you. Here lies the free choice of every human being.* One must realize, however, that one has to work, in the meantime, on **the "true" healing** of an ailment — that the FUNDAMENTAL HEALING of an illness will only take place when one **realizes** and **solves** its FUNDAMENTAL CAUSE: and that happens on a deeper level than the purely physiological or chemical. That actually happens on the emotional and psychological levels, in the realm of emotions and convictions, of expectations, and of the image one has of oneself.

I am not interested in "convincing" someone; I only offer deep, called-up Information, and everyone has a free choice either to use it or not. I consider it my task to write down this received Information and place it at the disposal of all good people.

Finally, let this book function as a "Key," but don't cling to it. Go onward, live yourself, and be your own master. Never cling to a signpost. You can only make grateful use of it in order to more quickly get upon *your* track of life.

In the *First Part* of this book — completely revised and enlarged in comparison with its first English edition — I describe the liberating philosophy according to which I experience life. From out of the depths of my heart, I wish you, too, a wonderful, truthful existence filled with love!

Christiane
Ostend, 6 June 2001
Nazareth, 31 August 2009
Lierde, 21 January 2013

CONTENTS

FUNDAMENTAL ORIGINS AND SOLUTIONS FOR ILLNESSES

MEMORANDUM

THE KEY TO LIVING IN HAPPINESS

●

To arrive at *true* happiness, it is recommendable that the human being follows the *"Signposts of Life."* It's about *signals* that want to make something clear to the human being. Everything has its meaning. Life does not allow itself to be pigeonholed; everything is in motion energetically.

What, among other things, can be considered as *signals?*

- Pleasant as well as less pleasant **occurrences and happenings** — in the individual sphere or on a world scale. Why do you attract them (often unconsciously)?[1]

- **Foodstuffs**: why do you have an appetite for fruit or chocolate and why do you hate fish, for instance? Your spontaneous food preferences can teach you a lot for the sake of your welfare and personal development.[2]

- **Encounters with animals**, in reality or in your dreams: what is the essential symbolism of a specific animal such as a dog, a mouse or a bear?[3]

- **Emotional, psychological conditions** . . . : the why of anxiety psychosis, sadness, depression, etc. How to consider these states? How to achieve inner tranquility?[4]

---

[1] Read more about this in *The Signal Book.* This work has not yet been translated into English at the publication of the present book.
[2] Read more about this in *The Horn of Plenty — Psychological, Symbolic Meaning of Foodstuffs.* This work has not yet been translated into English at the publication of the present book.
[3] Read more about this in *If Animals Could Talk* . . . . This work has not yet been translated into English at the publication of the present book.
[4] Read more about this under the respective categories of *The Key to Self-Liberation,* as well as in *The Signal Book.* The latter work has not yet been translated into English at the publication of the present book.

- **Diseases and other phenomena**: the body speaks a language. Learning to understand the why of illnesses and other psychological or psychosomatic phenomena, and giving them a fundamental solution, belong to the most important building stones of the House of Bliss.[5]

BECOMING AWARE
About the Underlying Origins of, and the Fundamental Solutions to, Illnesses

First and foremost, it is important to realize that it is best for humanity that no "dogmas" or fixed rules are established. It is best for us to allow Life to speak for itself: Truth shows itself and doesn't need "a name."

The time has come that the human being learn to listen to that which Life asks of him from within, to that "voice of truth" deep inside himself, to that which "truth" — inherent to Life — wants. And that the Human Being now realizes that he has, in his own hands, the full responsibility for his life and shouldn't place it "outside himself." Yes, that his life lies completely in his own hands: that he will obtain INSIGHT into "how" life really functions, and that this will ultimately give him a yet unknown feeling of freedom and joy.

Then he will see and know how only he, the human being, can lead himself toward illness and misery or toward health and happiness.

And hasn't he yet realized this? Has he lived "unconsciously" through ups and downs, convinced that everything happened to him "just like that"? Or was he convinced that a power "outside" himself determined his life? Now he will gain insight into the fact that every human being, unconsciously or consciously, "attracts" every circumstance in his life himself. And therefore it is good for him to tune in as consciously as possible to the Voice of Truth inside himself and lead his life as consciously as possible with trustful and positive expectations regarding Life.

---

[5] Therefore, the book *The Key to Self-Liberation — Encyclopedia of Psychosomatics* was written.

In this way he will experience that "illness" or "recovery" isn't something that "just" happens to you — that illness is a signal, sent from deep within one's own inner life center, and that recovery occurs when one understands "why" this or that specific illness manifests itself, when one listens to what the Source of Life asks the human being to "change" in his existence. The more consciously the human being lives, and the stronger he tunes in to this inner voice of truth, the sooner he will "understand" his illness and the sooner the recovery process can take place. At least, when he puts the "received insight" into action, when he truly psycho-emotionally, or on another human level, corrects his course, there, where his Life-Core asks him to make changes.

It needs to be emphasized that no-one should feel guilty, inferior or mediocre because of his or her illness, and that illness does not mean a failure, a punishment or an expiation. Not at all. Illness and recovery have to do with evolution, with becoming more and more deeply aware. This doesn't mean either that someone who develops illness as a signal would be "a less evolved being" than a person who is "healthy" at present. It is always about continuously taking steps forward in the development process of the human being; this happens in a different way in every human being.

Illness is just a "symptom" of something that lies much deeper

Every illness is a "symptom" of something that lies much deeper; every illness, no matter if it is flu or AIDS, is a "signal" that something is going wrong on the deeper psycho-emotional level (that means going against the life current). Every illness has its origin in a much deeper level than the purely physical. It all germinates very deeply inside the human being and finally manifests itself in the body: the body speaks "a language." The body voices, brings out, that which inwardly is going "well" or "wrong."

Illness has nothing at all to do with "guilt" or the "punishments of god"! The body speaks the language of that which constantly forms it, allows it to exist, brings it to life, and maintains it: the language of the Inner Life-Center or the Highly Individual Self-Core, the driving motor of Life . . . present in every human being!

Fundamental Healing
Insight and Responsibility

That which we call "Original Medical Science" is the science that searches for the true "origin" of illness and therefore considers the cure as a realization and understanding of the psycho-emotional origin on the one hand, and offering a solution to it, on the other. If cause and solution are being sought on the *true* level where illness germinates . . . *then* we can ultimately speak of *fundamental* healing. If one occupies oneself with only observation at the surface, however — when one studies merely bones, muscular tissue, blood vessels, etc., "in themselves" — then one disconnects the deeper Human Content, the psyche, from the physical Body, and will never arrive at TRUE healing. In this case, one is able to temporarily fight "symptoms" and cure illness superficially separate from the Content, but sooner or later the Life-Core of the apparently "cured" human being will again develop yet another disease. This is in order that the human being will finally come to the realization: time to look deeper inside yourself.

Of course, scientific research is very salutary to humankind. It is of incredible importance. However, as long as one maintains the "division" between body and psyche, one can never arrive at *fundamental* solutions. Fortunately, the cooperation between conventional medicine and the psychological approach is growing slowly but surely: hand in hand.

There is a reason that you "get" *this* specific illness and not another — that it is not your friend, but "you," who are being infected with this or that virus. Yes, because on a deeper level — INSIDE YOU — there is a psycho-emotional condition that is ideal "fertile ground" for *this* virus. And your friend, who is not at all afflicted with this (unconscious) problem or this "psycho-emotional field," that is so typical of this virus-vibration, is therefore not being infected.

The same goes for all kinds of "illness": for instance you can only develop leukemia[6] — as a baby or as an adult — when the deep-rooted psychological field that is typical of this disease is present in you. Then your deepest life-center speaks the language of: "You have Leukemia, you have to solve something specific in yourself on a deeper level." Do it. And recover also fundamentally as a consequence. . . .

---

[6] The text about the psycho-emotional origins of leukemia is in *The Key to Self-Liberation – Encyclopedia of Psychosomatics*.

Never feel "guilty" about this, but understand in a warm and loving way the "why and wherefore." Never blame yourself, nor point at someone else because of his or her "illness," but always remain in LOVING UNDERSTANDING toward yourself, toward others. Every human being is in a state of evolution, in his or her own way.

It's amazing how our Self-Core pushes messages "outward," manifests them via the body in "signals": SO THAT WE MAY CHANGE SOMETHING in our existence, in order to become happier people. Seen from this point of view, illness is *sometimes* a "necessity" — it forces you to consider that to which you may have been closing your eyes for a long time, or which you unconsciously didn't want to "see" in yourself. It forces you to look at how you, as a human being, hinder yourself from going through life in a TRULY HAPPY AND MEANINGFUL WAY. In order to bring you toward "True Life" — via a healing process which has to go together with essential inner changes that will "beneficially" alter your life.

Living according to Truth — from out of Yourself — means Happiness and Health

"Truth liberates": every human being can work out for himself which path or life-philosophy gives him the most liberating inner feeling. The human being may come to the realization that he has "free" choice between following the path of "Life-Truth-Joy-Love-Trust" on the one hand, and the track of "decline and death - delusion and appearance - lies-anxiety - lust for power - covetousness-doubt" on the other — a choice for Good or Evil. This choice, and the deeds that are in accord with it — will determine whether the human being ultimately will become "truly happy" or not.

Therefore, it's important that the human being open himself up to "truth," to "goodness" — to Insight (becoming aware), to the Inner Heart (Love): all this in the full Belief that he, himself, can direct his own life, either toward misery or toward Joy.

The more the human being becomes aware that *he* has the say over his life — as long as he is open to information of truth and "does" something with it — then the stronger and sooner he can make himself healthier and happier.

This book, therefore, offers you Information, without postulating any "dogma" whatsoever. On the contrary: this Information urges you as reader inside yourself and offers you facts about which you can thoroughly ponder, if you like.

Supposing the human being lived completely "according to truth." Then, he would be an extremely happy human being. *The goal is that we get tuned in more and more to that which "Life" itself, Life inside of us, wants — to that which we can call pulsations of truth within ourselves — so that we may become ever happier as human beings.*

If we evolve in the direction of what Life — in conformity with the deepest truth — longs for, if we connect ourselves with it and act accordingly, then we will not only become ever more harmonious with ourselves, but we will also see an environment (creating it consciously or unconsciously) that will correspond with the atmosphere of happiness deep inside us.

This is a fundamental law of life. A law of nature: Man, work Consciously on yourself, on your own happiness, intensely attune yourself with the Truth, with that which Life inside you longs for . . . then you will not only raise yourself toward more peaceful, intensely happier atmospheres, but will do the same for part of the world.

The Conscious Choice
Life-Force and Counter-Force

The Life-Source, which is fundamentally powerful and eternally giving, bearing, and creating, has allowed a duality to exist within its womb, two movements that we could call "good and evil," "life-giving and deathly-destructive-taking," "directed toward truth and turned toward appearance / lies," "Life-Force and Counter-Force." Here, the elements mentioned first are each time on the same line — the same goes for the last-mentioned notions.

The human being has been given a free will in order to choose between Life-Force and Counter-Force (the anti-life-path). Only via experiencing, and becoming conscious of, this contrast between good and evil — truth and lies, life and death, joy and sadness, love and chilly egoism — can the human being come to the realization of what TRUE LIFE means: a CONSCIOUS CHOICE is being asked for . . .

It's exactly through *confrontations* with lies and appearances, with sadness and death, that the human being comes to full understanding of the Value of pureness, of joy and of Life itself. That he can come to a *sense of gratitude* because of the life inside himself. And this sense of gratitude then leads toward a greater feeling of Happiness, through which (be it unconsciously) happier circumstances in life are being created. Once a human being has made this fundamental Choice in favor of Life, truth and goodness, then he can start to build an existence that will bear happiness. Even though the voice of the Counter-Force in himself might come to the surface once in a while, he has resolutely made his Choice, with a strong belief. Now Life will assist him.

Living in Harmony with Life

Living on the wavelength of Life or living "according to truth" means that we listen to the deepest voice of truth in ourselves, to our authentic nature, to our Heart, to our *true* disposition. "**Living according to truth**," "**living according to Life**" asks you to be faithful to yourself, to your inner core, your pure source; it asks you NOT to listen to a small selfish, superficial voice, a voice that takes into account only narrow-minded rational or external factors — that which "should be so" in society but goes against authenticity, genuineness; or that which the human being absolutely wants to push through or sustain at all costs, or certain "generally received," fossilized and destructive rules, or that which others or society expect of him while he ignores his own inner voice of truth, his heart.

The human being who lives in accordance with Life does not sacrifice himself to anything or anyone. No, the Life Source does not ask this. Martyrdom and sacrifice mean just the opposite of Love. But this also needs to be understood in the light of the spirit of the times.

Evolution, becoming aware, new insights, awakening will always grow further. One should not hurt oneself, not sacrifice oneself to "others," to "society," to one's image. For this is a form of self-betrayal, a betrayal with regard to Life. The human being who lives in harmony with

Life does not allow himself to be led by desires[7] and greed, nor by egoistic patterns of thinking and living.

Doing good to others while fully **understanding** everyone's nature. No criticism but communication. Inner peace, no war. Gentleness toward yourself, toward others. Believe in the strong powers of creativity that are in you and go onward!

Listen only to the most elevated voice, the most noble feeling that is present in you. Here, one can quote the words: "Not my will, but Thy will be done." These can be interpreted as follows: Not that what the small "I" wants may happen, but *what the great voice of truth, the voice of Life inside yourself asks you.* Growing towards: I AM. I LIVE IN LOVE.

You can feel very well what that means when you entirely open yourself up to "truth," with receptiveness and love. When also you let go of "the absolutely wanting to have" and attune yourself to the richness of your BEING. When you are attentively open to the signals on your path. When you let go of everything and everyone, letting them "be" the way they are. When you resolutely take your life in your own hands without persistently fixating on anything. When you profoundly listen to that deep Father-Mother-Voice (which is YOU!) in yourself[8]: you, as a Nature-child who represents Life, tune in to the Good, to Truth . . . and you will see, sense — do what you feel you have to do according to this vibration of truth, and you will be happy. *Feel,* from out of your heart; allow inside you that flow of life: truth lets itself be seen and felt but you cannot possess it. Do not lie to your own deepest feeling, your intuition.

High morality is now inherently present. The human being who lives according to goodness will never "violate" his own nature, not even to please someone else, because he knows that he hurts not only himself — that Life itself is betrayed — but that by keeping alive a vibration of lies he doesn't help others either. In short: the world is not helped at all by this.

---

[7] See the remark about the use of the word "desire," on page 8.
[8] Read more about this in the third chapter of the fairy tale *The Twelve Gates of Prince Sirius.* This work has not yet been translated into English at the publication of the present book.

"Living in harmony with Life," doing that which your inner life-source asks of you, also means the following.

Rest when you are tired. Come into action when you feel the energy bubble in you. Drink when you are thirsty, eat when you are hungry. Listen to the feelings of your heart; don't live just as a rational robot. Do good to others, but first, completely recognize yourself in Self-Love. Don't sacrifice yourself to others, to an ideal, to a work, etc. Giving is okay, giving in love, but do not exceed your own limits. Dare to say "no" when deep down, you feel you have to; this has nothing to do with selfishness but with the deep feeling of truth inside you.
   Do not laugh when you feel like crying; do not live according to the conviction that you always and invariably "have to" smile. Be true and authentic. Do not live according to appearance; do not put on a mask. Enjoy the pure, beautiful Being.

"Living in harmony with Life" also means that the human being allows the shape of his body to grow from his heart, out of love — not according to norms imposed by an ignorant society where "wanting to have" and "desiring to please" are often put at the center. For this path ends in death.[9]

"Living according to Life" signifies so much more than described above. This is explained in other sections of this introductory first part of the book.

When you live according to Life, not to decay, then you also wish to understand the signals that you meet on your path. For instance, the deeper meaning of illnesses and occurrences. "Why?" What can you learn from them? How can you make yourself take a step forward through them, on your true, healthy path of life?[10] You don't offer resistance to understanding their deeper meaning nor to fundamentally putting into practice the solution.

You live in gratitude. You put the Heart at the center.

---

[9] Read more about this in the chapter *The Cult of Looks and Appearances.*
[10] Read more about the deeper meaning of all kinds of diseases in *The Key to Self-Liberation – Encyclopedia of Psychosomatics.* The deeper meaning of other "signals" will be discussed in *The Horn of Plenty, The Signal Book,* and *If Animals Could Talk.* These three works have not yet been translated into English at the publication of the present book.

No one can Possess Truth, but you can Attune Yourself to the Vibration of Truth, the Frequency of Life itself

In many books written in our world we can experience that they are not tuned in to the frequency of truth. There are certain things written that are in accord with the truth, but other things are completely small-minded-rational (cut off from intuition and feeling, from deeper knowledge), or are just imagined. These are not always written with bad intentions, but they are still misleading for humanity.

Other writings are thoughtlessly "copied" from old (sometimes falsi-fied) sources and are not even understood the way they were "then" intended.

Half lies, half truths: it is good for the reader to observe all writings *critically,* and especially to connect with *his own inner feeling of truth* in such a way that he can separate the wheat from the chaff.

This book has been written to offer information to people who con-sciously want to progress on the path to more joy and health. No one can "possess" truth, neither I nor you. Still, it is possible to connect yourself — while being completely honest with yourself — to what I call the "vibration of truth."

In normal daily life this means: live always in total honesty with your-self — without lying to yourself; this implies doing certain things or precisely not doing those things, saying certain things or precisely not saying them, manifesting or behaving in a certain way, not lying to yourself or fooling yourself; not trying to escape certain things con-cerning yourself. Don't hold up a mask, but show your "I" the way you really are inside.

This is very important, and many people live "in lies" or "in appear-ances" without being aware of it (because they ignore the "signals" sent to them by Life as warning messages). The final result is that they make themselves sick and unhappy.

Others lie to themselves very consciously. They are then not "faith-ful" to themselves, to the living voice inside themselves, to their own deeper, natural disposition. They have betrayed themselves and are raping life inside themselves, with all the consequences.

A Concrete Example

"A" visits a certain person and after just a few minutes he feels, deep in his heart, in his total being: "I have to leave here! I don't like being here. . . . Yes, I'm doing this for my partner, or for this child, or for some host, or to please a sick person, or out of pity — but really deep inside myself, I feel how life calls to me: 'Go, get up!'" But what does this human being do? He lies to himself, sacrifices himself, thinks it is not proper, or that it is impolite, or not "dutiful" and . . . uneasily remains in his chair. The next day, he has a headache and nausea, he's itching all over, and his back is aching. . . .[11] This is because he wasn't in charge of his life, but placed certain things ABOVE Life, above "Living according to Truth," above Love for himself. Things like: "That's how it ought to be," Propriety, The Rules (unnatural, artificial Rules), The Strict Duties (which curtail every natural freedom of a human being), Pity, etc. In so doing, he does not only lie to himself, but also to the person he visits. He places himself completely at the bottom and doesn't listen to his inner voice of truth. It is possible that another person in the same situation might feel good, doesn't force himself at all, so that it's not harmful for this other person to remain seated, as long as he feels that it is good for him.

It's important that the human being not place ANYTHING above his inner voice of truth, which is the voice of Life within him. This Love for oneself is something completely different from "trying to force one's own will," or "egotism" or being ungenerous. On the contrary. Love of oneself and egotism are two opposite principles.

Pity: with this, you don't help another person. You do help by being full of understanding and sympathy, possibly looking for a solution together. But, above all: by BEING YOURSELF IN TRUTH. Do not suffer, do not suffer with others, but be an Example of Joy, of Honesty and Harmony: with this you also help others. If you are honest with yourself and act according to true Love for yourself, then you will stimulate others to search for Love of themselves and truth inside themselves. Even if there sounds a loud protest, it's only through honestly being yourself that you serve yourself, Life, and others. Don't live ac-

---

[11] Read in detail about the psychological origins of these symptoms in *The Key to Self-Liberation – Encyclopedia of Psychosomatics*.

cording to the conviction that life asks for sacrifice, that you have to force yourself in order to please others. That doesn't help yourself or others to get one step ahead. In Love and Understanding you live "according to truth." And other loving people will understand you. If your behavior is not being understood or accepted — in this example, when you stand up and leave — then you are dealing with a person who "demands" or "expects," in other words, "desires" something from you. Although this is understandable, it is not really directed toward Life. This person should start to search for self-fulfillment, for love of himself, for gratitude, and should learn how to let go (of person A).

When you really feel inside yourself, when the living voice inside you comes rushing up, as it were, and says, "Go onward!" then get up from your chair, say good bye, follow this honest voice, and don't resist the inner truth. When you feel, "No, I'm lying to myself if I don't get up right now!" then don't try to stay glued to your chair because of rational or other ideas like "Tradition says it has to be this way," or whatever. Or because of lying to yourself, do you perhaps get "backaches" or "shoulder pains" that indicate you don't build your life on that straight-arrow, Honest Central Pillar of a Spine in you? Do you instead "hold on to" old habits that go against life (lying to yourself), and as a consequence do you feel heavy burdens on your shoulders?[12]

Moreover, when you remain FAITHFUL to your honest inner voice at every moment in your existence, then you do help not only yourself, but also others. When you live in HARMONY, with Love for yourself, and in this way listen to that voice of truth inside you, then you act according to truth and you send, perhaps unconsciously, energies of truth to others. In so doing, you unconsciously stimulate others to work on themselves. There is an interaction of honest energies. No matter how much the other person whines in order to hold on to you, or even emotionally blackmails you, do what you inwardly feel you have to do with Love for yourself. As a consequence, it's automatically good for the other person that you go away, even if he or she doesn't realize it. You cannot do "good" to others if you don't first act with Love toward yourself. This is the sounding of the bells of life: "Love your neighbor as yourself."

---

[12] Read more about the shoulders and the spine in *The Key to Self-Liberation – Encyclopedia of Psychosomatics.*

Action according to Truth always causes a positive, energetic reaction toward yourself as well as toward others. *You stimulate the truth-energy in others by honestly listening to the living voice inside yourself.* By placing nothing ABOVE this voice of truth. In this way, you help Life and the World along. Truth liberates yourself, but also helps others — when being confronted with your honest action — to live according to truth. . . . In fact, in this way this Love for yourself brings about a loving deed, also with regard to others, although they might not even be aware of it.

Being Faithful to Your True Nature

Another example: "living according to truth" means also *being Faithful to your True Nature.* If by nature you are round or heavy and robust like a farm horse, and you are in perfect health,[13] but you think you should look like a thin racehorse and you start to follow a strict diet, then you violate your nature, then you lie to your own constitution in order to answer to the exterior norms or rules of the society in which you live, a so-called slimness-ideal — or whatever certain people think they have to promote as being the only healthy way, (because they are convinced of it and follow the indoctrinations of society). Here, too, the same rule applies: Listen to your true nature, in Love for Yourself. *True beauty, health, authenticity and truth lie on the same line.* Someone who is falsely thin — e.g., by losing weight just for looks' sake, or by following a strict, narrow diet — will sooner or later have to pay for this lie against one's own "I." Sooner or later, this false "beauty," this Appearance will crumble.

What counts is to be plump or thin in a healthy way, small or tall, so that the form is an honest reflection of your NATURE OF BEING. Things go wrong when the human being begins to doubt his Power, his Mobility, his Natural Being. *No matter what your body shape is, when you live out of true Love toward yourself, with the conviction that you are strong, mobile and healthy, then your body will grow in health.* **On condition that you "live in harmony with Life," of course!** Please read the chapter about this point earlier on in this introductory part of the book. Everyone will move through life in a way that honestly sprouts out of his nature of being.

---

[13] as has been confirmed by medical examination (e.g., blood tests).

It's the same regarding the practice of sports. Taking physical exercise is generally good for your health, but if you practice a certain sport while you really don't like it, against your nature, then you lie to yourself. Just FEEL, very deeply inside yourself, whether it is something for you. Especially listen to that voice of truth inside you. And even if you receive useful information from others, you yourself "know" best and "feel" best what's good for you. Listen to your heart, to the "signals" on your path.

As a rule, it's good for your health to take exercise. But what kind of exercise? Running is good for whomever likes to run, biking is good for whomever likes to bike, swimming is good for whomever likes to swim, etc. But as soon as it becomes an "obligation" or an artificial, Spartan "course of treatment" by which you force your body, then something is wrong. Then you listen to rules that are imposed on you and possibly do not at all correspond to your true nature. *Never do something that makes you feel: "This does not correspond to my physical nature, my constitution."* Do not "hurt" yourself. Don't ask a "rabbit" to cut trees, and don't ask a robust person whose job it is to fell trees to do excessive jogging. Do only that which you feel is in harmony with your true nature. Read more about this in the chapter: "The Cult of Looks and Appearances." Yes, it is healthy to keep moving in a joyous and relaxed manner — not under stress or under pressure to achieve.

Do you eat things you actually don't like just because it is supposed to be "healthy"? Then, you lie to yourself. Trust your nature, as a human being who lives consciously and transforms his instincts into consciousness energies.

Do you pierce your face with holes, do you bind your feet, do you lace up your waist, or do you carry out other painful rituals because "that's how it should be" within the tribe, the community, the country? Then, you place rituals, behaviors, external things ABOVE Truth, above Life. This cannot be salutary. Dare to question everything. Arrive at love for yourself and know that the ONLY true health and beauty can but go hand-in-hand with the "truth." This means that your body grows from out of love for yourself, that it radiates beautiful love; this has nothing to do with the so-called norms of beauty that reign within a certain society. Bodies that are formed — consciously or unconsciously — according to these false norms within society, detached from inner love, are fake, unreal, and therefore ugly (although one often does not realize this anymore). Sooner or later this results in illness and deterioration. After all, lies destroy themselves.

"Signals" as Road Signs on Our Path

Sometimes, we don't realize we are lying to ourselves, or that we are not completely on the right Track, not completely connected with the honest Stream of Life. Luckily, there are Big Signals and Little Signals that draw our attention to this.

It is necessary that the Human Being learns to live in the "here and now" in a Conscious Loving way, and learns to look at Signals on his life's path so that he can adjust his course where it is beneficial — first of all for himself and, as a result, for all of humankind. By "Signals" is meant: illnesses, emotions, circumstances that arise, occurrences, experiences, etc.

Less pleasant situations or painful Signals, like certain *illnesses, are there to show that we are more or less deviating from what Life in us intends. These Signals ask us to adjust our life's course in order to arrive at more joy and health*. And these signals don't just appear out of the blue. We — unconsciously — call them up ourselves. After all, Life inside us wants to bring us farther and farther along on the way to happiness. It is us, ourselves (be it unconsciously), from deep in our Life-Core, who call up Signals in life in order to make something clear to ourselves: "Somehow, you are on the wrong track. Correct yourself, so that you become a *really* living, happy, healthy Human Being."

Frequency of Truth

In order to write down my texts I tune in to truth frequency. I "call up" the texts in a concentrated way, after which the answer is received very clearly and consciously from the depths of the source of truth. Therefore, the calling-up and writing-down of *The Key to Self-Liberation* — which includes the deepest psycho-emotional causes, the actual initial phases of about 1,000 illnesses — happened very fast. Within a time span of less than half a year, *The Key to Self-Liberation* was written. It has nothing to do with the observation of illnesses or sick people, nor with reasoning out or study, nothing to do with mysteriousness, trance or channeling, but with a very clear tuning-in to a deep inner knowledge. The human being has really no **need** for "guides, angels or extraterrestrials" in order to advance in evolution. Although I respect everyone's opinion and actions in this matter.

Every Human Being Has Talents

Every human being on this earth can feel that immensely powerful life-source deep inside himself; everyone has his talents, his possibilities, his specific task. It is, for instance, important that someone who has the talent to make furniture uses this talent in order to make people happy with solid, pleasant furniture. And when the baker who succeeds in baking delicious rolls thinks he *has* to come to a state of enlightenment by doing something else (although he experiences so much joy in his work) then there will be no delicious rolls on the shelf, and he is wasting his time with things that surely will make him feel "No, this is not my task."

Life asks that every human being, true to himself, do what he feels he has to do according to heart and soul, in joy for his earthly "I." One task or job is not worth more or less than another. And every human being will open himself up to what his Living Self shows him to do or not do.

The greatest talent is "TO BE" as a Human Being, in thankfulness. He does not "want to HAVE" (things or people), he is not a slave of desires.

And all together, consciously living, good-hearted people, we contribute to the construction of a New World where it's good to live: here on Earth. It is better that we don't pay too much attention to the negative (without sticking our heads in the sand, however). Instead, let us bring building stones for that which is pure, honest, and New. **Evil cannot but destroy itself in the end. Good will strengthen itself and multiply**. And Life goes along with the frequency that corresponds best to its aims — so that, from out of our Living Self, which is full of love, we can know and say that the delicious-beautiful, the Good, will ultimately triumph on Earth.

The Meaning of Life . . . is Life itself: Living-in-Love; The Human Being experiences his "I Am" in the ultimate Happiness to then share this with other people

It is of utmost importance that the human being, in his search for the meaning of life, for true happiness, in his search for "truth," dares to question everything — but really everything — that ever has been presented to him as being "truths" or "lies," whether through his upbringing, religion, political-philosophical, mainstream or alternative schools, etc. The ideal attitude of the consciously seeking human being is critical openness and "receptiveness" full of trust, while throwing overboard every "prejudice": He does not "just" accept anything without questioning — like a zombie — does not just discard anything in a prejudging way. Neither does he think anything to be "impossible."

This is the most honest and healthy attitude of the human being in search of the "truth," of the true meaning of Life. A healthy, critical, though open approach to everything he hears, sees or reads.

It is necessary that, in his search for the purpose of Life, for the "truth," the human being is able to build on a fundamental certainty, an unfaltering principle, which serves as a basis. There is one basic truth, one certainty, running as follows: "I-AM-HERE-AND-NOW." This observation, coming from the human being who lives consciously, doesn't need further proof. There is no basis "under" this basis. It serves as the Basis of Certainty to this human being who can know, feel, and be aware. Very important is this certainty: on this basis, the human being can build his life as an unshakable construction, in a never-ending growth-process.

Believe in Yourself!

Here, it is very important that the Human Being come to a greater awareness of his "I," that he develop a strong Faith in himself, in his "I." After all, one of the greatest causes, if not often the deepest cause of misery and illness, globally as well as individually, is a lack of Faith in one's own "I." It's necessary for the well-being of a Person that he comes to a greater Faith in himself. Faith goes hand-in-hand with becoming more Conscious.

The human being is a living being . . . it is therefore necessary, in order to believe in himself, that he first and foremost chooses in favor of Life, believes in Life. And, finally, that he fully becomes aware that he, as an "I," does not "just" exist here, without any reason: every human being is the realization of one of the endless, profuse expression-possibilities of Life itself, and *every* human being has at his disposal highly individual, unique possibilities, *far* more than he suspects!

Every human being has actually formed himself within life's womb, however unconsciously, and from the beginning has always driven himself onward on the basis of an inner, unique disposition that grows and grows and grows.

Life has sought its path, ever further, and finally has put itself into the world of matter, bringing itself to further realization in "the human being." The human being is the result of a longing by Life to see itself reach a higher level of fulfillment; for this goal an alliance is formed, in a concentrated way, between the physical and the energetic, spiritual (consciousness energies) in highly unique beings. Man should realize that, inside himself, he has at his disposal all possibilities to function optimally as an autonomous and original being; that in himself all possibilities of Life are there, allowing him to make himself into a healthy, happy being: as "himself," and not similar to anyone. The wonderful spectrum of the enormous diversity of people spread over the Earth.

There will be only misery as long as the human being allows himself "to *be* lived" in an unconscious way, and doesn't bring about CONSCIOUS changes where they are needed for his well-being: changes in his expectations and convictions regarding his existence, in his "passive" way of living, in his disbelief, etc. It's now up to the consciously living human being, in his shaped uniqueness, full of Faith in himself, to bring "Life" further along — to help "Life" progress. It's up to the human being himself to unfold his energies, his possibilities, and to direct his life, full of confidence. We would say to everyone: "As a Human Being, take your life ever more consciously into your own hands. Bring yourself to realization. Believe in your own uniqueness. Begin to search for 'truth,' and listen to that honest voice of Life in yourself."

Every human being has that choice: Are you going to allow others, or exterior things, to rule you, letting yourself droop, living according to the conviction that life is a vale of tears over which you have no say? Are you slipping into a "depression," which by itself is already a signal that you need to change your course, that you don't consider Life completely "in accord with truth"?[14] Or will you, on the contrary, start to live according to the conviction that you can make of yourself someone who takes deep delight in everything life offers, simply by listening to that voice of truth in you which teaches you that Life is something marvelous as long as you yourself contribute to its creation?

The voice inside you that gives you the most true joy is the LIVING voice, because real Life and Joy go together. Therefore, don't listen to a voice in yourself (thoughts, convictions, etc.) that brings you sadness, because this voice is called "lies" and goes directly against true Life.

Take your life in your hands, make something wonderful of it!

Do you notice that you become "sad" when you think of the past? Then stop this thinking and resolve, from out of the Present Moment, to experience the most beautiful situations in your life.

You Create your Future Yourself, Consciously or Unconsciously

Every human being creates his life himself, consciously or unconsciously. You create your future yourself . . . there is no question of predestination, of fate or destiny, or of karma having to be paid off, of punishment, etc.

The way someone's life, someone's reality, someone's future, unrolls, is the result of one's deep, embedded expectations, convictions regarding oneself and life. Are you convinced that you deserve punishment or that life entails suffering and victimization? Then you will experience sad circumstances and possibly "attract" an upbringing or dogmas which confirm your deeply embedded expectations of life. Why are you convinced you will have to encounter punishment and suffering? Is it because you are convinced you are a "bad" or "sinful"

---

[14] Read more about depression in *The Key to Self-Liberation – Encyclopedia of Psychosomatics*.

person? Then it is to your advantage to start seeing yourself as a good human being and live accordingly . . . drawing a line through the past. Then you will attract beautiful life circumstances.

Know: *you can start every day with a new, clean slate, whatever your past might have been,* as long as you have the honest, sound intention to be good, to do good. However, as long as you remain convinced that you have to do "penance" for sins from a "previous" life (part of life) then you deviate from the Voice of Truth inside you which represents Life; this voice just wants to stimulate you to start again as a Good human being, NOW, today, and no longer hurt yourself because of possible mistakes or feelings of guilt from the past. So, stop burdening yourself with karma and original sin. "You as you" can, indeed, start anew every day, in goodness from out of your heart.

The word "sin" can be described as a negative conviction that you have put upon yourself and on the basis of which you have begun to live and act. The most important "sin" the human being has put upon himself is: Doubt in the "I," in one's goodness, in one's abilities to create one's own life. A doubt which often goes together with a kind of discontentment, dissatisfaction, unthankfulness. Doubting "whether Happiness on Earth is possible"? This conviction is so deeply ingrained in humankind, from generation to generation through the ages, that we can really speak of "original sin." A deeply rooted conviction of Doubt that has already inflicted many wounds.

It's time now that the Human Being, in thankfulness for his existence, in Contentment regarding his "I," no longer doubts his ability to create eternal Happiness; that he no longer doubts his divinity, his Goodness. If he eliminates this self-degradation, this deadly *Doubt Virus,* then he will no longer feel the urge to fill himself with greed, desire, militancy, apathy — then misery, war and illness, and finally physical death will disappear.

In other words, the "fall" of mankind (as described above) has indeed been a painful transition, and this is still the case of most human beings. But it has its value for Life if the ultimate result is "The Faith in one's own Power and Goodness." If suffering and death are once and for all banned to the past. If Grateful Contentment triumphs regarding one's own existence! The resurrection of Life in every good Human Being on Earth: for ever. Eternal happiness on Earth is possible if the Human Being believes in it and lives according to truth, to Love, in a Conscious way.

The things that happen in your Life show you which deeply ingrained convictions regarding yourself and regarding life you were born with; why you unconsciously attract certain situations; these may be always situations of the same nature, again and again. This doesn't "just" happen by accident. Occurrences, events, emotions, but also illnesses, are being called into life by your "Living Self," your "inner core," in order to make something "clear" to you; in order to make you realize where you as a human being cause yourself pain, where you lie to Life inside you.

The deepest living and life-giving principle inside you (which I call the "Living Self") constantly sends out signals; because Life in you wants to bring itself further along, via your existence as a unique Human Being, in a highly individual, honest and positive way. In other words: YOU as "I"-THE-HUMAN-BEING want to bring yourself, in a highly unique way, further along the path which will lead you to an ever-greater consciousness, to happiness. That's why the Living Self sends you signals again and again. Especially if something happens that goes directly against life. Then your Living Self sends you signals. Look, then, at these signals. Do not try to nip them in the bud; after all, looking at and understanding these signals can bring you, as a Human Being, a big step further!

The future is not "predetermined"

Sometimes we hear people say: "Everything that psychic has predicted has happened." If the future is not predetermined, how then is something like this possible?

The answer is: by NOT believing that the future is "not" predetermined; by living according to the conviction that everything in the future is predetermined, and that one cannot change it anymore. The "fortune teller" doesn't see "THE" Future of the person concerned, but sees the person's expectations as they are projected toward the future "by that person's convictions." When these convictions (especially of an easily influenced person) are, in addition, accentuated by the "predictions" of the psychic, then it's not so surprising that this person — who, on the basis of his convictions, creates his own future — will create a future that coincides with the predictions. The psychic then helps to "determine" a certain future. The important thing we can say here is: the fortune teller (without it being his first intention) makes the person aware of the deeply ingrained convictions that dwell inside him.

For instance, a pregnant young woman came to tell me that "a certain psychic" had predicted she would bring a handicapped son into the world, and that her marriage after two years would run aground. And that everything "he" had predicted to one of her friends had come true. Her fear was great. After I explained to her how "predictions" work, she determinedly started to take her life (and future) into her own hands. Living according to the conviction that NOTHING negative needed to happen to her, because she lived according to goodness. She banned from her being every "negative" conviction regarding fears that had to do with the birth of her child and her marriage. The negative predictions about this person *NEVER* came to be.

Regarding "predictions" about world happenings it's not difficult to pick up certain *unconscious* "streams" that dwell among humanity and "to see" a future on this basis: however, when the Human Being (as part of humanity) arrives at unexpected new Insights, and on the basis of this brings about Conscious changes, then these unconscious lines "turn" as it were in a new direction. Then, no single prediction about the future will turn out to be correct anymore. Then, reality makes, as it were, a "curve" that no fortune teller had foreseen. THE FUTURE really lies completely open. Therefore, it's of utmost importance that we, as Human Beings, become aware of deeply ingrained convictions in ourselves, in order to transform all of them into happy, optimistic EXPECTATIONS of the future! Every human being will experience that which he consciously or unconsciously has created *himself*. Therefore expect THE GOOD . . . and live accordingly. Don't get into a panic when certain less-pleasant occurrences or symptoms pop up as a "signal": look at them and make adjustments as needed. Believe in it . . . and everything will work out fine!

Illness as a Signal

Illness is not something that "just happens" to be unalterably spread over mankind, as a result of which some are met by good luck and others by misfortune. Illness is a symptom — from the flu, to AIDS, to decline, to death — a signal that your Living Self-Core sends as a warning in order for you to thoroughly realize something, and to change your existence. To make you become "aware." In other words, you are doing something that doesn't run completely in the direction of "Life," because of which life cannot completely and optimally stream through you. Depending on how and in which way you need to adjust your life-convictions and deeds, you will develop this or that ailment or illness. Depending on what kind of "deviation" from Life you maintain in yourself — thoughts, convictions, emotions and actions that go along with them — you will attract this or that illness.

So, for instance, someone who has developed a throat infection[15] has not listened to the voice inside him which asked for an honest expression of emotions, asked for autonomy, for emotional independence from others, and especially for him no longer to bottle up sadness and anger, which often go together with desires and demanding things from others, with feelings of rejection. Imagine that someone doesn't at all listen to the "signal" of throat infection and that this throat infection finally disappears, with or without medication — but surely without working on the psychological causes of throat infection; after a while the infection disappears because the psycho-emotional causes have "eased off" or are being suppressed (but are not fundamentally resolved). Then this person can after some weeks or months develop the same illness, or perhaps bronchitis[16] . . . Why? Because his Living Self now sends out an even stronger signal in order for this person to finally reflect on the question of what Life inside him really wants. Imagine this person allows his bronchitis to heal just by taking medicine, or by whatever alternative treatment, *without working on the true psycho-emotional cause, Origin, of this ailment.* Then his Living Self again will send a signal, possibly even stronger than bronchitis . . . so that he finally might listen to himself, to the "why" of this illness, of this signal. And one, therefore, should not be surprised that Life ultimately brings forth illnesses like pneumonia, cancer, etc., as signals: in order to still offer the human being the chance to take a better look at this more serious signal, in a conscious and in-depth manner. In this way, the *fundamental* psychological solution can be realized (simultaneously with the possible medical treatment).

---

[15] Read more about the symbolic meaning of this ailment in *The Key to Self-Liberation – Encyclopedia of Psychosomatics*.
[16] Read more about bronchitis in *The Key to Self-Liberation – Encyclopedia of Psychosomatics*.

Because humankind is often keeping itself ignorant; because most people regard illness just as a symptom (at the most call it sometimes psychosomatic); because the human being never looks deeper into the *true* causes of illness, into the *true* origin (there, where the illness originates, there, also, originates the healing process!). That's why Life itself sends new illnesses again and again, illnesses that are ever more difficult to "suppress" or "heal" with medicines . . . so that the Human Being might finally start to look deeper into the *true* meaning of the signal called "illness." In this way he can become aware that illness as a symptom, as a signal, is there to show the Human Being another way, indicate a better life . . . a life that connects with the stream of truth and therefore with more joy, freedom, happiness.

Illnesses that are more and more difficult to heal, like AIDS,[17] are for the human being to really start to reflect now, in a healthy, conscious way; for him to consider the possibility *that the fundamental "healing" of AIDS or whatever illness doesn't happen on the level of medicine, but on a much deeper level.* The human being, *every* human being, has his own healing process in hand much more, as long as he dares to look at the reason, the true causes of why he has attracted this or that ailment. Once he has understood this well, he can recover from this "signal," this symptom, this illness, by putting into practice what the signal (illness) asked of him, by bringing about changes in his life. Taking medicine is okay, but at the same time, one needs to take a deeper look into oneself.

Humankind, and also "medical science," may and can no longer neglect these signals from Life itself, from the human being himself, if it wants to progress. When will medical science begin to search for the "True Origin" of illness so that we can call it "original," and "truthfully exploring the depths"? Fortunately, numerous doctors over the whole world are enthusiastically responding to this work and often report in delight that "it really does work that way!" Doctors, health professionals, and laypersons who are searching for "truthful information," for "more in-depth information," and for "true healing." The time has come that educational institutions and universities make room in their curricula for health professionals in order to help them arrive at deeper insight into the true "origin" of illness.

---

[17] Read about the psychological undercurrents of AIDS in *The Key to Self-Liberation – Encyclopedia of Psychosomatics*.

At present, medicine, surgery, etc. are still necessary for humanity. You can make use of them, provided you work at the same time at solving the underlying psychological pattern. One cannot dissociate the body from the psyche, the emotions, the spiritual consciousness. Disease and cure need a fundamental, global vision and global approach.

Trusting Your Nature. Convictions. Immunity

It's very important that the human being "lives from out of himself," that he believes in himself, that he honestly dares to be himself. But how many people put this into practice? It has been taught to the human being not to trust himself, his nature. "Don't go outside without a scarf or you will catch a cold." This is a conviction that indicates a view of oneself as a weak person and a lack of confidence. Certain people have a susceptible throat or neck by nature. They feel comfortable when they put on a scarf. Well then this is a gesture of love and honesty toward one's own body.

But this is something completely different than, for instance, the person who by nature has no susceptible throat or neck and who lives only with the firm conviction that "he MUST put on a scarf when he goes outside, otherwise he will inevitably catch a cold" — even if there is no strong wind or cold temperatures. A kind of ingrained disbelief makes him doubt that going outside without a scarf will *not* cause him to catch cold.

Here, everyone will need to be faithful to the *true* nature of one's body. It is very possible that the person who lives merely with the IDEA that "he *has to* wear a scarf" will get very warm, too warm, during his walk. But he is afraid to catch cold . . . . He does not believe that by nature, he need *not* catch cold when he is faithful to himself and when he feels inwardly that his throat will not suffer from it.

However, if he develops this basic confidence and changes his convictions, then he BELIEVES that a scarf is not necessary for him. As he is faithful to himself, he also believes in his immunity. He loves himself. He does not live according to the aforementioned IDEA. Instead, he remains faithful to his nature. So, in this case, he does not need a scarf — that is to say, on the condition that he does not carry inside him all the psychological patterns that underlie a common cold or a sore throat.[18]

If in the following week it's comfortably warm, not even a breeze, not at all cold, but this person at that moment is psychologically very hard and cold toward himself, living in a rather deathly way, without warm feelings, as if wearing a mask . . . yes, then he can "catch" a cold, regardless his "trust," because the psychological field is very attractive to this specific virus. This person will heal from his cold by breathing warm life into himself, by coming home closely and warmly to his inner heart, and the Force of his Faith will very quickly help him over it.[19] The same or similar "scenario" we can quote for every illness.

Because the human being does not believe in himself, in his immunity, in his natural powers . . . he becomes more susceptible to illnesses. HIV/AIDS, for instance, gives a literal translation for the paralysis of the immune system. Now the human being, mankind, begins to mistrust its own nature even more. Because, who can still trust his nature if the immune system can be paralyzed by a virus just like that? It becomes a whole vicious cycle that the human being has to break through if he wants to purify himself from all the disasters in the world of illness.

Medical science, science in general, will have to study the true causes of illness in a very honest, open, conscientious way. Without doubt, when the necessary apparatus will be available, it cannot but find that every illness in its essence has its origin in convictions (do you believe in yourself, in your immunity?), and in the nature of the psycho-emotional field of the individual who develops a specific illness as a signal[20] . . . so that he might free himself of the underlying causes.

An important task of the health professional or doctor is to show the sick person the Core of the matter, the true underlying origin of his ailment, and to stimulate him to believe in the effects of self-healing forces (which does not mean that medicine as a remedy will have to be discarded right away; read more about this in other chapters).

---

[18] Read more about this in *The Key to Self-Liberation – Encyclopedia of Psychosomatics*.
[19] It is obvious that one has to be always honest with oneself. When, for instance, it's a raw day and you are cold, then it's normal that you put on a warm coat.
[20] Also read more about genetic predisposition in *The Key to Self-Liberation*.

Fundamental Solution

So, dear human being, believe in yourself and work yourself out of this pernicious cycle of self-doubt!

It doesn't matter if you take medicine or not, if you follow conventional or alternative methods of healing, make use of acupuncture or take allopathic pills — all this is not at all "bad" or wrong, but it has nothing to do with the CORE of the matter, nor with the ESSENTIAL SOLUTION of your illness. It can give you a kind of temporary balance, of comfort, a feeling of "being cured," but *true, fundamental* healing can only take place when one "works" at healing on a deeper level at the same time as the "treatment" — or without treatment, depending on one's conviction. There, where the illness once started, on a psycho-emotional level — on the level of convictions and emotional depths — when a solution is offered for the *real* cause of illness that lies hidden *under* the physical. By looking precisely at the nature of the physical symptom (illness) and understanding it, then we can arrive at such a thorough, permanent, fundamental healing.

This can only happen when the "patient" *opens himself up* to this true "cause and solution." Because then, after all, he has to take responsibility and begin to do it himself. It is much easier to resort to a "remedy" without working on the deeper causes. And this doesn't *have* to be done (working on the fundamental causes), except that the human being will have to realize that his Life-Core then soon will send him a new illness (or another signal), in order for him to finally begin to heal himself and make himself happier in his CORE.

You don't just "accidentally" become infected by HIV/AIDS or whatever illness. For instance: two people, one of whom carries the HIV/AIDS virus, can have sexual intercourse for years, without the other person becoming infected. This is because this person doesn't at all carry the inner psychological field that creates susceptibility to this HIV/AIDS virus.[21] I totally recommend the preventive use of condoms because the human being generally does not realize, does not know whether he is susceptible or immune to the HIV/AIDS virus.

---

[21] Read more about the HIV/AIDS virus in *The Key to Self-Liberation*.

We see a totally different "psychological pattern" with the flu virus[22]: when one person in a group of twenty only "infects" four of these people, it just means that the psycho-emotional field that is sensitive and susceptible to the character of the flu virus is present in these four people.

We have seen many people who have healed themselves from cancers, tuberculosis, rheumatism, etc. Certain ones took medicine during their psychological development process (healing process), others did not at all. Be careful and do not take any risk. Always act in consultation with a competent conventional doctor. In any case, fundamental healing demands you look closely at the reasons why your Living Self-Core has developed in you a certain illness as a signal. A solution for the underlying psycho-emotional causes is necessary. As a result, healing forces are being stimulated, the immune system is being invigorated, and consequently the human being also heals on a physical level.

And whether the human being takes medicine or not depends on where his conviction begins and ends. If he is *rock-solidly* convinced that it is possible to do without, and if he *really* does what he "must" do on a psychological level, then he will heal in that way.

However, most people have not yet arrived at this degree of personal development; therefore they should take no risk at all and not become reckless. (And moreover they should not allow themselves to be influenced by the possible recklessness of certain health professionals who consider themselves more capable than they really are.) **If there is anxiety, or the person does not dare to be without medicine, chemotherapy, operations, or whatever, then it is best that he does make use of these things.**

But, a complete and lasting cure on a fundamental level depends on the psycho-emotional evolution which one carries through inwardly, at the same time as the conventional medical treatment. It is important that the human being should love himself, arrive at Insight into the *true* cause of his illness, "work" at it, believe in himself, in his self-healing energies.

And no matter if it's about an ordinary cold or HIV/AIDS: it's always about "signals" from the Living Self. If one has understood them well, then one can thoroughly work on the essential solution and, therefore,

---

[22] Read more about flu in *The Key to Self-Liberation – Encyclopedia of Psychosomatics.*

on the healing. This is, actually, the only *true* healing — when one deals with the fundamental causes of illness-symptoms and pulls them out by the psycho-emotional root. The "signal" coming from your Living Self-Core was understood, and the necessary changes were brought about. This is true healing. But don't feel yourself to be a "failure" or a psychologically weak person when you avail yourself of medicines, surgery, chemotherapy, etc. This is a good thing.

The person's convictions play a very important role. Imagine that someone heals himself from a severe ailment through — as he expresses it — following a diet, or by taking this or that miraculous herb or medicine. Then, on the one hand, this is the result of this "diet" and these "herbs" or "pills" interacting well with the SYMPTOMS of the illness. On the other hand, it's the result of the fact that there is also a back-up from the strong **conviction** that asserts "This diet and these herbs or pills are going to heal me." And the person heals . . . apparently. Another person with the same ailment, who follows the same "healing method" doesn't heal at all from the "symptoms," because his conviction doesn't back up the healing process. But, in reality, neither has "healed fundamentally," because they only look for the solution OUTSIDE themselves.[23]

Sooner or later the Living Self will send a new, possibly more severe, illness to the person who heals himself SOLELY on the basis of help from the outside *without looking at the real psycho-emotional causes, his own deep-rooted convictions:* an illness for which diet, pills or herbs don't work anymore. This then happens in order that he will start finally to look at the deeper, *true* cause of his illness, in order that he will become AWARE, in order that he will TRULY bring himself to healing.

Therefore, never ignore the message from your Living Self-Core — *whether or not you take medicine or herbs, whether or not you let yourself be operated on. In the meantime, don't forget to work on the REAL REASON for your illness. In this way, you will come to true (inner!) healing. Therefore, as a result of this, your body will no longer have to attract any other severe signals.* Although I saw in my life many cases of so-called "unexplainable" miraculous healings, I am grateful for the existence of, for instance, conventional surgery. Dear people,

---

[23] It is for this reason that one should never reproach the doctor / health professional / surgeon in attendance.

if necessary, *allow an operation or another radical treatment to happen, with love toward yourself, without feeling you have failed, without feeling guilty. All in good time. In the meantime work on the deep-seated cause of why ever you attracted this tumor or whatever as a signal, and then . . . your Living Self never again has to develop such an illness. Because you have "understood," because you have changed your life in the direction the illness asked for.* Believe in yourself, in Life, in those fathomlessly deep life-forces which exist in you. Love yourself and don't close your eyes to the Insight into the true cause of a certain ailment. In this way, you will finally heal yourself of minor and major ailments, if they still would happen to appear on your path — possibly without help from the outside. But don't rush anything, don't take any risk. Be *thankful* for the existence of conventional medicine when, or as long as, it is necessary. Therefore, do not reject it.

With illness as a signal, always question yourself: *"why" THAT illness, THIS ailment?* The Key to Self-Liberation explains the specific psychological-emotional origins of this or that ailment. Don't ignore this. Also look at the minor signals, like headache, a sore throat, a small finger wound, etc. — so that your Living Self-Core doesn't have to send "bigger" alarm signals to you later on.

A good example is *eczema:* if you don't listen to what this skin ailment wants to tell you, and you don't do anything else but suppress it with creams, pills, or herbal products, then we sometimes see how the same person who was, allegedly, "healed" from eczema, now starts to suffer from asthma.[24] If you don't bring about the psychological changes the signal "eczema" asked for, then your Self-Core will call up an even stronger signal to force you to work thoroughly on yourself and so bring yourself to fundamental healing. There, where eczema, among other things, calls you to greater recognition of your spacious energy field, asthma will even more strongly reflect how you experience yourself as anxious and empty. Therefore, search for your Fullness, the broad space of your being, etc.

You don't *need* to suffer pain. Pain is a signal the Living Self sends out to make it clear that you would do good to take up your space in a

---

[24] Read more about eczema and asthma in *The Key to Self-Liberation – Encyclopedia of Psychosomatics*.

fuller, larger, and more loving way, and that you are "hurting" yourself in certain areas. And, as a result, you attract pain, accompanied or not accompanied by an illness symptom.[25] *Work* at the deeper origin of this pain and illness . . . and, yes, if you have the feeling that it's necessary, take a painkiller. Life allows this — on the condition that, in the meantime, you work on solving the causes of this pain. If you don't do this, then you are just suppressing, ignoring, the "signal" that your Living Self sent you in order to urgently bring about changes in your existence. Listen to this. Be gentle to yourself, but go onward, bring about changes where it's necessary.

And then — as we[26] have seen in practical life, when someone has gained insight into the psychological origin of his pain and needs few, or no more, painkillers — pain will just disappear if that person does what life asks of him, for his own well-being and transformation.

The same is true for *anxiety and depression* (read more about this in *The Key to Self-Liberation*): the human being can do without medicine, but it can be good to temporarily use a remedy from the outside, even if, in principle, he can do without it and has everything within to imme-diately make a turnaround that will cause every anxiety, panic or de-pression to disappear, as long as he believes enough in himself, car-ries love for himself inside and shows willingness "to change."

But, in reality, we see that certain people need some time to get rid of old resistance, to find a new track, and then it isn't "bad" or "unhealthy" to temporarily find a remedy in this transitional phase. One doesn't have to have any feelings of guilt about this, as long as one doesn't misuse remedies from the outside: here, too, it's only good and justi-fied toward Life in you when you at the same time work on the true psycho-emotional solution, when you bring about necessary changes in your convictions, your actions, etc. — when you "let go" of old things. If you are convinced that you can get by without remedies from the outside, so much the better.

No matter how you do it, arrive at honest, fundamental healing, via the faith in yourself. Resolve this undercurrent so that happiness and har-mony will become an ever-greater part of you.

---

[25] Read the text about "Pain, in general" in *The Key to Self-Liberation*.
[26] I and the doctors with whom I cooperate(d)

Emotions as Indicators

"Emotions," too, are signals from our life-core. Also, the less-agreeable emotions need not be considered negative, but should be regarded as important indicators.

Do you feel **sadness**? Then this means that you deny an important part of yourself, of your essence as a Human Being, and that you insufficiently acknowledge your worthiness and your creative forces, the thankfulness for your Being. Listen to this . . . and help yourself. Believe in your inner greatness and offer yourself love. Life within you wants nothing more than that you are in constant "JOY"!

Don't forget: a certain happening in your existence is, in fact, only the **occasion** for a certain emotion, such as anger or sadness, to come to the surface. Then, it seems as if the cause of your anger or sadness lies in those happenings. No. **The cause** lies much deeper: solve it deep inside yourself. You have already carried a vibration of anger inside you, and as a result you have attracted a situation in which you get angry, not the reverse. In this way, happenings and your emotional reactions to them, can reveal that anger, anxiety, sadness, feelings of guilt — or whatever emotion — are still to be found in you. *The circumstances you unconsciously attract are only a result of the emotions already existing inside you.* Look at them and bring about changes in yourself so that you come to a greater harmony within yourself.

It is precisely thanks to the occurrences which awaken a certain emotion in you that you can become aware that this emotion is (still) present in you. This then allows you to get going and transform this disagreeable basic emotion into pure joy.

When someone gets into a fight then it's because the fighting spirit and the aggression were present in him beforehand. It is not the mocking laugh of the other person that brings up his fist — *this is only the "occasion"* — it is the deep-seated feeling of anger, powerlessness, anxiety in himself, the auto-destructive mocking laugh toward life in himself. These are the *True Causes* through which he attracts such a situation and through which he begins to fight and furiously uses his fists.

Christiane Beerlandt®, Life Philosophy – © Beerlandt Publications, Lierde, Belgium

Is there still **anxiety** dwelling inside you? Then once in a while you will attract situations which, allegedly, will "give" you anxiety. Know, then, that anxiety is a signal from your Living Self to make something clear to you. "You have to adjust your course in order to arrive entirely upon the path of life and happiness."

Some examples: Do you give yourself too little love? Are you suppressing your formidable life energies? Do you constantly sacrifice yourself for others, or do you cling to them? Are you only living on the superficial periphery of yourself? Are you constantly keeping your thoughts in negative spheres? Or are you on the track of discontentment, greed, and desires? Then, anxiety will be awakened in you . . . in order for you to realize: in this way you can never make yourself happy; this path leads to death instead of life. Therefore, be thankful that your Living Self-Core makes you feel anxiety in order for you to become aware! As soon as you have solved the basic cause of anxiety, in love toward yourself, then you will no longer attract situations which will give you anxiety.[27]

Hatred. Every feeling of hate toward others finds its roots in hate toward Life itself, in the inability (or resistance) to UNCONDITIONALLY love Life and your "I" with regard to form and content. Therefore, don't put conditions on life. Experience your unique, beautiful Being in Total Love of Self, in thankfulness for Life itself. Hatred toward Life also means that you feel discontented and unthankful, because you don't have or can't get "this" or "that" the way you would want to. However, if you arrive at unconditional surrender to "Love for Life," and "Love for yourself," then you tune in to the vibration of BEING, and no longer to the wavelength of WANTING and coveting. Then the current of life can flow, unhindered and happy, through your veins. This happiness for who you are, for the fact *that* you are allowed to exist "as You," without placing any other conditions on life, results in you attracting circumstances that make you happier and happier.

Also, with regard to **traumas**: you mostly place the cause for your misery in some happening from the past, whereas that happening was already a result of an inner "atmosphere." You then have attracted unpleasant situations — be it unconsciously — in order to look at the deepest cause, the "why." Why, what energy field lives in you so that you have created such situations in your life?

---

[27] Read more about anxiety in *The Key to Self-Liberation*.

When you arrive at absolutely clear insight regarding this, then you will look at the past with different eyes and will no longer place in others the cause for why this happened to "you," but will place it in *yourself* (even though this doesn't mean that the behavior of the other person can be justified). You will bring about changes in the PRESENT, and ultimately you will look at the past in a detached, liberated way. In this case, it doesn't make sense to keep stirring it up and follow reenactment therapy for years.

A spontaneous outlet for emotions is, on the other hand, natural and healthy and belongs to the psychological digestion process: no matter whether you are alone or with friends, or whether you have a good understanding with a doctor or therapist — ultimately you have to, and can, do it *yourself*. It is certainly okay to have a healthy communication with someone, with a health professional. You can pick up interesting information here and there, through teachers and books, but ultimately you, yourself, remain your own "chief professor." Count on yourself, and know that the solution of whatsoever problem is inside you! You can do much more than you think, independent of "help" from the outside — which doesn't mean you cannot have helpful talks with others without, thereby, falling into a position of dependency. It's important to allow yourself to express certain emotions, to let them flow out, very spontaneously, and not bottle things up. In a next phase you begin to search for the "why," for the causes of your discharging of fury, sadness, hatred or whatever feelings. The deeper **causes**, the roots of these emotions, you always find deep in yourself; the circumstances, happenings, people — these can but be **occasions** through which these emotions "surface." In this way you can lovingly allow yourself "to be," "to evolve," to better understand yourself.[28] It doesn't make sense to stimulate emotional discharges in a forced way.

Live from out of your heart and trust your nature, your feeling. Consciously be your own Leader! Trust that intense, self-healing powers are present in you.

Life, itself, doesn't want anything more than to allow its "emotion" of Joy to flow through you without being hindered . . . so attune yourself to that life-giving source inside you, listen closely to the signals on your path, and — full of trust — go onward. In this way you will get there for sure!

---

[28] Read more about emotions in *The Key to Self-Liberation,* as well as in *The Signal Book* (which has not yet been published in English at the publication of the present book).

Desires

"**Desires**," greedily "wanting to have or to possess," are also signals. If you look closely at the object of your desire and understand this, this is also a means of bringing yourself into greater harmony with Life

By nature, the earthly human being is a wonder of power and fullness and vitality. **But because he doesn't believe enough in his power, value, and fullness, he has given existence to all kind of powers and forces outside himself, which have to replace, as it were, the forces and values that he denies in himself**.

The human being who believes in his own powers and lives from out of himself, autonomous and full of love, experiences himself as a "fullness" and feels the true joy of life flow through him. Inside himself, he has disposal over all the possibilities of making a paradise of his existence on earth. When, however, through a shortage of faith in himself, he projects his powers, his contents, his possibilities outside himself . . . there comes about a feeling of missing something in himself. The human being no longer feels "complete." True joy no longer flows.

Deep inside the human being lives that longing to (again) have that feeling of "fullness"; he starts to long for what he misses inside himself, because he has placed it outside himself. Desires represent, therefore, a longing of the human being who doesn't experience himself as "complete," a longing for a state of "completeness," for a state of joy that he naturally can experience in himself.

According to that which we desire, we can find out *what* we still keep outside ourselves, what we miss in ourselves to feel complete. An example is the urge for power. A person who's plagued with this has little or no mastery in and over himself (or an aspect of him); this urge will diminish according to how much that person develops mastery over himself. See also further on, the chapter about Power and Manipulation.

When desire is directed toward money, then we can look at what money symbolizes. This person has to deal with his self- respect, with the true values inside himself. He will need to value the material (physical) aspect of himself.

Do not follow anyone but Yourself

Something more about **power and powerlessness**. Certain people who possess special gifts (like bending metal objects without touching them, performing magic tricks or materializing money or gold, or changing or moving objects in an inexplicable way, or healing illness symptoms through magnetism) often feel they are called to say "it" to others. They bind others to them and feel good in this position of power;[29] certain sect leaders, for instance, attract people who want nothing more than that someone else, preferably someone they look up to, will lead their life. In this way, power and powerlessness meet each other: both sides hold on to each other in a situation that is not exactly directed toward life.

The only thing these magic-makers prove is that the human being has much greater ability than he suspects. (Magnetism and so-called paranormal gifts are not necessarily parallel with the state of awareness and the degree of love present in a human being. Sometimes, there are unwise and loveless "leaders" who gain power by showing off some of their tricks or by charming others in a sweet way.) In the meantime they need to realize that their longing for power and leadership over others is a signal from their Living Self to strive after more power and leadership over themselves. The "followers," on the other hand, need to realize that they'd better break with a conviction and feeling of powerlessness, that they only need the faith in themselves in order to step healthily into life in all freedom and joy. Often, certain charismatic people keep others in their grip in a subtle, emotional way. We cite here the well-known words: "Ye entered not in yourselves, and them that were entering in ye hindered. . . ."

Therefore, we repeat again: **believe in yourself, as a human being; believe in that formidable life-power that is present in your inner source, your core; believe in your highly unique individuality, in your ability, and take your life in your own hands! Don't follow anyone but yourself. If you like, enter into dialogue or relationships with others, share your love if you like, but never lose mastery over yourself, over your life. Make something beautiful of it, you as the masterful, loving leader over your existence.**

---

[29] It's obvious that not all "miracle workers" act with negative intentions; things are put strongly in the text only because there are so many abusive situations.

Your Living Self Exults

Every human being is born within / out of the womb of Life. (By many, this Life Source is called God.) In EVERY human being there is *a primordial Life-Core* present which "wants" (by an inherent drive, wanting to see itself fulfilled) nothing more than that the human being attune himself to True Life: that he will bring himself further along in life, and grow, create, produce, evolve, *feel,* blossom, so as to make Life *itself* progress in this way.

In this sphere of life there exists no (self-) degradation, no death, no drawing back or in . . . **only giving life and life-growth**. We call this element, this life-stimulating power center in the human being, *the Living Self-Core:* present in every human being in a different way (because every being forms itself from within in a highly unique way), but there is always one common point in all: as individual manifestation of the primal life-power (the 1 detaches itself from the 0, is born as "I") moving itself forward in the direction of Life

The Living Self-Core wants to concretize itself, as optimally as possible, in a specific, individual bodily form that is appropriate for this or that person to allow to live — experience, develop in an infinite way — his life, his task, his talents, his enjoyments. An honest manifestation in "matter," in the body. *The Living Self* then represents the total human being, who as "content in physical form" truthfully exists as a "living Unity" and longs to "Live"! So, the Living Self that is you, YOURSELF, as far as you are tuned in to that true Life-voice according to "content and form."

The soul center, "deepest self," or Living Self-Core incarnates itself in a REAL, honest and pure, physical body, not in a sham body; this is a false body that is created by the Counter-Force in a human being — the "deadly" force; a body that is artificially built up, inwardly molded, manipulated in order to want to please, seize, impress, draw in, have power, seduce, attract, etc. Instinctive sex-energies draw the fly into their web, as it were. **If a human being identifies himself with this "mask" — with the external, superficial side of himself — then he gets completely lost, distancing himself from his *true* Essence; then anxiety and panic can arise and finally death, as the ultimate disease.**

So, every human being can listen to the honest Life Force in himself or . . . to a kind of Counter Force, an anti-life atmosphere. Every human being has to make this choice. "Happiness" or "misery" are inextricably linked with this.

You can either connect yourself with the atmospheres of the Life Force or the Counter Life Force, the Anti-life force that works against, blocks, or would like to kill life. **If you attune yourself to the Life-stimulating atmosphere inside yourself, then you will automatically grow, will transform instincts into consciousness powers, and begin to live more awarely in greater love**. And if you sometimes make a mistake — listen to the atmosphere of anti-life — then you will immediately attract signals that will indicate that you are no longer on the track of Life.

You are "you" with your consciousness-content, with your highly unique nature in the physical body that is you and which you form from out of your Living Self-nuclear-force. The body in Unity-alliance with the content: an intimate contact, a feeling of joy is the result.

Automatically, when the human being connects himself with the true voice of Life in himself, he won't sink to "lower regions," to a sheer animalistic, instinctive life, to greediness, etc. In this case, he will ultimately no longer experience anxieties and sadness; after all, he continues to search ever further for his inner source, his inner greatness; he unfolds his potential powers, his abilities, in goodness. Finally, he bans every illness, all suffering, even death. That's the ultimate goal of the life-giving Power Sphere that is present in every human being.

Illnesses are signals of our Living Self-Core, to show us that we are not yet completely connected with Life; if we evolve further, listen to these signals, and do what life asks of us, then the ultimate illness (the physical dying) finally will no longer be needed at all as a signal.

There's always the possibility present in the human being to listen, on the one hand to that which we call good, noble, high-minded, connected with true Life, divine, the most beautiful and loving elevated spheres, a pure consciousness level unsoiled by maliciousness or greed . . . pure values of being, etc.: the voice of our Living Self. On the other hand, the human being can roam in the spheres of what we call darkness: the egotistical, vain, undirected toward Life level, the

Christiane Beerlandt®, Life Philosophy – © Beerlandt Publications, Lierde, Belgium

energy which kills and demands, self-denigration, the image-oriented, the small "I" which undervalues and denies itself in its greatness, remaining stuck while doubting goodness and truth, in spheres of destruction and self-destruction, of animalistic sex-without-love, of decadence and death.

The human being always has the CHOICE to ennoble himself, to attune himself to the first voice inside himself (it isn't literally a voice one can perceive, but rather an inner sphere or state of being). This voice directly connects with Living according to goodness and truth. It is that in the human being which connects with the powerful, Living energy-flow. We call it The Living Self, because it is so totally in harmony with Life itself. When the human being tunes in to this Choice, to these spheres that are directed to life, then he experiences true Joy and Love; then he opens himself up to signals and new information which will guide him farther on the path of Life without end.

What matters is that the human being opens himself up to this feeling of truth, this voice of Life deep inside himself. And, if he cannot "reach" it very well, then that is because he has fixated too much on the exterior of his being, or on his outer appearance, or, for instance, because he has been "thinking" way too much — no longer *feeling* — or because he was completely convinced that nothing was there under the superficial layer of the human being, under this "thinking above all, and maybe feeling and sensing a little." He has strayed from his inner being, from his vigorous, driving, vital force — the engine that propels his life ahead — by focusing too much on the "outer world," on appearance, on image, on others. He has closed himself off from his inner riches.

It often is asked: "**But how do I reach my inner 'Life-Core'? I can't make any 'contact' with it.**" Many then begin to search in an anxious and panicked way for "something" that should be there. No! That's not really how it works.

First of all, you experience *your body*. If it is not being manipulated to gain power over others (through seduction, drawing in, attracting, impressing others, etc.), then your body is an honest manifestation of your Living Self-Core! If you experience your body, feel it, see it, *feel* intimately and lovingly connected with it, then you *are* actually (in this body) your Living Self! Of course, there are "unconscious regions," but you don't have to direct yourself to them. You *know* that in the sphere of soul and body, your Living Self is being driven by an infinitely powerful "Life-Core" inside you. For the rest: tune to *your HEART,* to Love, to giving to yourself — and, as a result, also to others — to intense and sincere receptiveness to what Life inside you asks of you (and, of course, to *doing* what life wants you to do), to feeling your earthly, living body. Then, everything will become clear to you through what you *feel,* through the signals you encounter on your path. Feel your heart, love your body, because in this orientation toward life "YOU" *ARE* YOUR LIVING SELF! Even if you cannot reach certain "underlying" regions, this isn't necessary at all. Direct yourself deeply inward and, there, *profoundly sense your warm Content;* don't get hung up in "outer" spheres ("How am I being perceived?") but *live spontaneously from within.* Be who you ARE!

Let go. *Live* joyfully, live according to your heart, to what you feel, your intuitions, using your common sense. Consciously follow the signals on your path, trustfully, not fanatically — and then you know that you *live,* that you yourself are your Living Self at body and soul level.

Your Living Self is not something that is hidden very deep inside you; you don't have to dig a thousand miles under the sea! Tune in to your heart, to love, feel your skin, your honest body . . . the Word of Life was made "flesh": this is real, living flesh. Open yourself up to that which the inner life wants of you . . . and you will feel it. Just OPEN yourself up to what you see, hear, and feel, and to what the essence in you that is tuned to true life (your Living Self) attracts as signals on your path. And, if that Life-Core, that powerful "engine" in your being, drives and directs you further and further, don't then fight *against* it. Go along with yourself and never abandon life in yourself by clinging with your superficial small "I" to certain things or people or false values. Listen in all honesty to what inner life tells you, to your heart. *Let go, and go further onward* in an eternal, happy growth-process.

Finally, dearest Human Being, take up your Inner Kingship!

We don't *allow* ourselves to "be lived" by "Energy," by this complex totality, by this bulwark we are, by the 1001 rich facets in us, **but we Direct our energies ourselves, very Consciously and lovingly.** We don't have to "comprehend," know, all that goes on in deeper, more unconscious layers of our Living Self. But we may realize that the Potential in Powers is enormous; this asks for Leadership!

Christiane Beerlandt®, Life Philosophy – © Beerlandt Publications, Lierde, Belgium

Allowing that, under the impulse of Love and Insight, animalistic, instinctive energies transform themselves into noble, highly human consciousness energies, directed Creative powers. *The "male" and "female" aspect, in balance, united* under the supervision of the Conscious leadership of a loving "I."

A being-open, in receptivity to the unconsciously living content and wisdom deep inside us. Ever keeping the balance between heaven and earth, between spirit and body. The brain will function optimally, and its capacity regarding "knowledge" and "awareness" will grow when the human being takes his place Consciously at the head of the Living Unity he is.

The Crown on the Living Self: the human being as Master over his existence in wisdom and in love. He rises above the narrow-minded rationality and listens to the *true* wisdom that lives inside him. Every human being has the ability to do this as long as he doesn't begin to "cling to" or "greedily fixate" his "thoughts," or his "emotions," with an urge for power, and is attuned to the truth-frequency of Life. *He lets go, and allows himself in all spaciousness TO BE,* taking up his task as Leader over that multitude of conscious and unconscious life-energies in his being. He makes his way *in trust,* and he *knows* that everything will be all right.

To Survive or . . . to Live?
Physical Immortality?

The human being has been living for so long with *the conviction* that he has no other choice than eventually to die. You can ask yourself: and what if the human being no longer lives according to this conviction? It is a fact that Humanity knows itself to be imprisoned in "the web of life and death" and that it has created consoling perspectives to escape from this concept. And then came the answer, from the very deep source of truth, the most beautiful I ever "heard" — described under the title "New Days."[30] The path to physical immortality now lies before the human being who is open to it: however unbelievable it might sound, it's about a choice and the consequences of that choice, *the consequences of reversing deeply ingrained convictions.* Physical

---

[30] At the time of the first publication of the present book, *New Days* is not yet available in English.

transformation follows that inner choice, inner transformation. *Every human being is free to believe what he wants* and to determine whether or not he will make this or that conscious choice. Nothing is compulsory! Follow your Path. Here, I can only say that this liberating philosophy creates completely new, joyful perspectives, and once you are on this path of "Life," it will strengthen and enormously uplift your faith. However beautiful you might imagine life after death, I am talking here about death and dying as the ultimate disease to be overcome — in goodness and elevated, powerful faith.

Follow your path[31] the way you feel that it will bring you the greatest happiness. But in so doing, don't forget the altruistic question: on the one hand, what will best benefit Humanity as a whole as far as being-happy is concerned and, on the other, what can expel anxiety and sorrow?

The Image of God

Most people on our planet worship a certain "Image of God." Because humankind did not believe in itself, it has projected its power and forces in divine images outside of itself. From the divine image we see, we can deduce what values this person or this race embraces. The human being really created his gods according to his deepest longings (or according to his greatest fears): so, too, has the human being who highly regards Love and "expects" this love also from others created a god who represents love. In this same way, the human being who admires toughness and strength, militancy and courage, has created a god in this image; he always expects trials of strength and only feels good in struggle. Thus, in the human being who created a god which has to be adored, celebrated, and praised, there lives the longing that he too might be acknowledged and adored by others, just as he approaches his god . . . . but, in fact, he has a need for self-acknowledgment. Thus, the human being has created an immortal god because he, himself, actually would like to be immortal (and deep inside himself he knows that he actually is); this indicates the deep longing to break through the age-old pattern in which he keeps himself imprisoned: "having to die." The god who demands obedience and

---

[31] By "you" is not meant the small "I," the ego, but your deep, inner, divine, conscious "I," which is full of love.

metes out punishments indicates that in fact the people who adore this god also expect obedience from others, and otherwise would possibly mete out punishment. But they, themselves, can also have the feeling that they are treated in the same way by their fellow men and — because they are hard on themselves — fear a kind of punishment.

So many people, so many gods. Therefore . . .

If we use the term "god," then — in order to get out of the worldwide confusion of tongues — it would be preferable to regard this as "LIFE" or "Life-giving Source" out of which everything has come forth. But we don't have to place anything or anyone "above" ourselves, or project outside of ourselves, because by doing this humankind immobilizes itself in powerlessness. Life doesn't mean powerlessness; on the contrary, this is the last thing in the world that the Source of Life intends. The more consciously you begin to stand in Life the more you will notice that you, and only you, consciously or unconsciously, lead your life, have it in your hands. There isn't a fate or commandment at all that stands above your head and will tell you what is good or bad. *The divine life-energy flows through the Hearts of all of us. It is up to us to steer this energy in a conscious manner.*

Live in Thankfulness . . . for Life inside you, in Love toward yourself and Life, in helpfulness toward Life. Follow the signals on your path; *your inner life source — or divine source, if you want, will show you the way.* But it's up to you to take your place, solidly and self-aware, at the head of your ship of life. Listening to the language very deep inside you, listening to and looking at the signals your life source attracts. Redirect, adjust your course and go on ever further on that path of happiness.

All the people in the world who are good of heart and honest, thankful for their existence, permeated by Love, and of pure Faith (in themselves and in Life!), can meet one another on *this* wavelength. Here, it no longer matters what "religion" they practice or have practiced or if they are without any religion. **Within the blissful House of Hearts**[32] **every good human being is welcome, a true "encounter" is possible**, because one no longer "hides" behind a system. Here dogmas, doctrines, no longer count; truth speaks for itself, shows itself in The Act of Life. Here, churches, mosques, temples, and other houses of

---

[32] Read more about this in the book *The Twelve Gates of Prince Sirius, the Ninth Land* (not yet published in English at the time of the publication of the present book).

worship no longer fight each other, *because every Human Being lives from out of his Good Heart, with Understanding toward those who live differently* — because one now realizes that such struggles for the sake of religion were just "alibis" in order to get rid of deeper, ingrained frustrations. Now, all buildings can be opened — for Life, for True Love, and for all people who don't place anything or anyone above this Heart. An encounter between "Life"-friendly people with built-in high morality, by which peace and strong faith in one's own ability to make something beautiful of life go hand-in-hand. After all, every feeling of powerlessness (and as a result urge for power), every defensive or offensive (war-minded) behavior, disappears with this deeper "Knowledge" of the "Ability" in every human being to create one's own life, directed by "Goodness" and by "Faith" in that inconceivably strong, pure, Inner divine Essence. *Peace, Joy, Understanding among all kind-hearted people . . .*

Love

Do you love *Life* itself? Have you chosen to firmly say "yes" to Life on Earth? Then, within this scope you can also love *yourself;* after all you offer yourself life, in thankfulness, and that is the most beautiful thing you can do. This *Alliance with Life* indeed consists of *unconditional love for yourself.* Sheer, pure, intense Love of yourself on a body and soul level: the way YOU are, unique and irreplaceable, authentic in form and content. You radiate this love of life, this joy for your existence, this love for your "I." It's about a state of "being." You allow your heart, your thymus, your brain, your entire body to be filled with thankfulness and love of Life and of your "I." *Then, it is honest and good to share this Love with others.* Then, you will also be able "to give without expecting something in return," unconditionally . . . without bartering: "I give you this if you give me that back!" The latter is, of course, not love. But also, self-evidently, if you live according to pure, self-radiating Love, and give with your heart, then you will automatically experience encounters with others that are full of love. (The reader can test this out for himself.) A generous, happy, radiating state of love simply attracts similar vibrations toward you: don't give in order to possess, to obtain, but *give* out of Love for yourself, for the life current inside you, in thankfulness for existence itself, for your existence, and for the existence of other good people . . . and you will turn yourself into a happy being. You will radiate this happiness to others, who then also will be stimulated to search for love and thankfulness for life, for love of themselves. Others will be confronted with their hate or self-hate; they will be stimulated to resolve this in themselves and to transform themselves into a pure state of love.

Often, the human being is born with certain "expectations" and "instinctive" tendencies. He needs to develop Love inside himself. Although in some people this inclination is naturally more present than in others, many people again and again "expect" everything — in the first place from their parents. It's good that a young person soon learns that *"giving" means "life and happiness," and that seizing, demanding, expecting only brings sadness, anger and a state of unhappiness.* He needs to learn that he will do well to take good care of himself — to offer himself love, in thankful contentment for existence, for what "is" there in his life; that it is necessary and good for him not constantly to want to possess and possess, falling from one discontentment into another, because desire creates new desires again and again. If things go wrong here, then later on he will project into a partner relationship the same demands and expectations and how his parents reacted to his behavior. The things that were not corrected in childhood are later on presented again as "lessons of life."
    Therefore: love for oneself, allowing the full heart to blossom, thankfulness for just having been given the privilege to live on earth, this attitude, this Feeling . . . makes it possible for this child or grownup to attract beautiful situations . . . which then make him even happier. It's a path of life full of joy, without end.

Love of Oneself does not at all mean Egotism

Love chases away every anxiety. LOVE FOR ONESELF is a great necessity for solving any problem. This has nothing to do with selfishness, with vanity, with egotism or image (these are accomplices of the counter-force of life), but has to do with true LOVE toward one's own total "I."
    Living in warm-hearted unity with yourself means allowing yourself to truly LIVE and no longer remain stuck in sadness, anxiety, old patterns that once again will lead to suffering and death. You offer yourself the Highest Love. You don't expect it from someone else.

You don't have to go and live on an island, alone and far away from all life. On the contrary, enjoy; pouring out pure nectar to yourself! Feel like a god in the earthly paradise; make yourself warm, comfortable, cozy. Do only what you feel you have to do from YOUR HEART. No longer listen to that dark voice; offer yourself a conviction of joy: be convinced that the Good is stronger than the Evil and then Evil and darkness will disappear by themselves from your conviction-sphere. Offer yourself the most happy, loving energy.

Love means *giving* . . . to yourself. And, as a result, you can also give to others. As soon as you begin to ask, to demand, to hold on to things or persons instead of to give, anxieties and dark, obsessive convictions can plague you. So, let go . . . give yourself Love. When you are tuned in to this high Love toward Life and toward your True Self, in Trust, anxiety will disappear.

Don't you acknowledge yourself? Do you pull yourself down or do you consider yourself just as a limited, small or ugly being? Then you don't yet love yourself enough. Then you may be anxiously holding on to old patterns, to the primal mother womb, to people or things outside yourself, which makes *a free life-current* impossible. And *then* your Living Self sends you anxieties and panic to point this out to you: COME INSIDE YOURSELF, in your blissful EARTHLY BODY; love yourself, no longer push yourself *away!* Don't flee from your true self; don't flee into thoughts, in the "spirit"; don't cling to old patterns, to "drugs" or to other people. And, if you listen to these anxieties without running away from them and replace these anxieties with faith, Love, pure love for yourself, strongly coming INTO yourself, in your body here and now, with both feet on the ground, fully present in yourself — then anxieties will ebb away.

The mother and the father are INSIDE you. Don't deny either one, but lovingly integrate these primal powers inside yourself. Count on yourself; offer yourself Faith, Trust, and Love. Acknowledge your worthiness as a human being, your deep inner worth — and love yourself the way life has given shape to you: you *are* in your body, the way you are at its best. Don't desire to create — out of thirst for power — another outer form; be thankful and content in love toward your body-form which is an externalization of your inner, unique nature. Throw overboard every power-norm and seductive manipulation. Don't draw others toward yourself in an instinctive way, don't be like a suction force that absorbs others, but *give* from your heart. Fulfill yourself. Don't put DEMANDS on life, nor on yourself; listen to the language of

Love. Then *give* to yourself, letting go of everything and everyone, also the old, compulsive patterns. In this way you become a fearless, happy human being.

True beauty and goodness are one and the same; they have nothing to do with *"sham" beauty,* which exists within a society that employs / indoctrinates false norms, disconnected from the heart. It's up to the human being to unmask this lie of appearances, blinding, and fake beauty. For this leads to death, it drags you along toward illness and pain.

The light of real LOVE FOR YOURSELF chases away every dark conviction, because true "love" will no longer tolerate fundamental sadness, suffering, or death to be present in your existence. So intensify this Love and be convinced that no single power is stronger than *this,* since it goes hand in hand with Life, with Goodness, with Truth, and even can bring Life constantly further along in its progress.

Living in Relationship, in Friendship — in Love and Happiness

Certain people like to go through life without a partner. They have every right to do so. Do you choose to live in a relationship? Then first and foremost work on the relationship with yourself, arrive at pure Joy about yourself — only then can you experience pure Joy in the relationship with the other person.

Relationship is *giving, not asking or demanding.* You don't **have**[33] a partner / a friend, you **are** a partner / a friend.

You, yourself, attract EVERY situation, good or bad — albeit often unconsciously. It is advisable to live "more consciously." So make something beautiful of it.

Do you have the feeling that the other person doesn't love you enough? Then this often means that you insufficiently love yourself. Offer yourself more warmth, more love.

If you seize and hold on, you will be seized yourself, by anxiety, sadness or, for instance, an obsessive urge for sex.

You can say or discuss certain things — for instance something you have on your chest — but then you let go of it. You don't demand, you

---

[33] Have = possess.

don't expect ANYTHING from the other person. You give, you speak and you let go of your partner. Then you come very close to yourself, ever closer, in profound contentment with yourself.

Thankful Contentment for life inside you. This thankfulness, this Love toward yourself, warms your heart. You say "yes" to life that is in you. In this harmony, this joy about life in yourself, you will AUTO-MATICALLY attract these things and human friends with whom you will go on the path toward "the earthly paradise."[34] Certain friends from the past might disappear from your life, because they are not on this path. Then let go of them, in peace. Learn to say "No," when you feel so. Go to certain people when you, yourself, feel like it, not because "someone" expects it from you.

In the feeling of thankfulness circumstances change; problems solve themselves — if you stop blaming others, stop having feelings of ha-tred or resentment, because your partner doesn't want to "fulfill" your longings. After all, with this discontentment, desire, this criticism to-ward others, you don't get anywhere; you will only make yourself sick. This "wanting to get something out of the other" lies on the path of illness and death. Therefore, let go of that other person. Come very close to yourself and transform hatred into love, criticism into thankful contentment for what IS there! And you will see how life rewards you; you become warm, comfortable inside, and relationship problems, too, solve themselves. On the basis of your love for yourself, everything that is good for you will happen. Let go, don't seize, don't grab, don't blame others . . . and turn inward. *Give,* talk things out, and let go, staying very close to yourself, which also makes it possible for your relationship and love toward the other person to grow.

Stand on your own basis. Live from out of yourself. Stay faithful to yourself and at the same time learn to understand each other. Let the past be a closed book in order to be there for each other in the present, shaping yourself in a New Form. Not selfishness, but love. Not losing yourself, no blind amorousness, but a strong concentration on your own Basis. Two people who live on their own strong basis can meet each other as equals. Everyone has his shortcomings, his strong or weak side to work on. Therefore, never point your finger at someone else, but always work on yourself. Then things will go well.

Don't lose yourself in someone else, because then you will be on the path toward death, where also blinding intoxication, empty ro-

---

[34] Full of peace, transformed, where happiness and justice reign.

mance, and sex without love belong. Therefore, be faithful to yourself. Don't do anything you really feel you shouldn't do, not even to please the other person, because then you lie to yourself, with that you don't help the other person either. Only the truth endures. . . .

Therefore, choose Life in Love, choose truth on the highest level. Work on yourself and, again and again, let go in order to discover yourself, down to the roots.

Leave the other person free, loose, because true Love is without Ties. Don't suffocate each other, give each other freedom. In this freedom there is faithfulness and a deep alliance. Wherever you are, no matter how much distance or time separates you from each other, in your heart you are always together. This alliance has a strengthening effect. In this happiness, you go on with YOUR tasks, and your partner / friend with his / hers. You are thankful and content because you are . . . in Life, because of the relationship which is allowed to be, *this* relationship or friendship which is best for you. And you trust your Living Essence and let go. In this way joy can flow through you. And you FILL yourself only with yourself, although your heart rejoices to feel the love for the other person flow through it. But first and foremost you have to love yourself, very deeply. Only then can you exchange this love with someone else. Otherwise you would do things that go against your own nature, and sooner or later this will take its toll.

Power-struggle needs to be avoided completely. No one is worth more or less than the other. Don't elevate yourself above the other, do not "tell" the other from above. You, too, have your faults and shortcomings. Always keep talking and living on an EQUAL level with each other, and calmly say what you have to say.

Don't try to bind the other person, to hold him/her tight to you, to pull him/her toward you; this is use of power. Give with your whole heart in joy . . . then everything will go well. Things go wrong when you end up in the lane of discontentment, disgruntlement. Therefore, be glad and thankful for the Life inside you and for that which *is* there. The rest will come at the right moment. Life will give you at every moment what is good for you. Don't seize, don't grab, don't demand, because it isn't always that which you think is good for you that is best. From out of gladness, the thankful contentment with your own Being — all happiness comes to you.

Do you feel anger, hatred, or sadness "because of" someone else's behavior or "because of" a situation, an occurrence? This means that these emotions are still deep inside you and need to be cleaned up if you want to be happy. Does a certain situation awaken sadness or hatred in you? Know, then, that you have attracted this situation as an *"occasion,"* so that you would solve the *"cause"* of this sadness or this emotion in yourself. So that you will come to pure joy and thankfulness for your being. Your happiness depends on you. So, come to warmly loving yourself in thankful contentment with life; then life will finally reward you. Come, in warm love, close to yourself; then you can *give,* not expecting anything from the other person, but fulfilling yourself and making yourself happy; and then you share this happiness with your partner or your friends, in a relationship that vibrates at the frequency of truth.

"Life, I am thankful that I AM" — and, in this feeling, you know that everything and everyone will come on your path the way it is good for you . . . so that finally you will be able to live toward greater happiness, in eternity. *Therefore, let go of everything and everyone outside yourself, turn inward very deeply and be thankful. Then everything will happen that is good for you and for your happiness.*

About Love and Sexuality

It's important to realize *that sex is not love, and love is not sex.*

Two people who love each other very much can, within the language of the heart, under the warm mantle of love, meet each other in sexual intercourse. But it is not a must. Certain people don't at all feel like having sex, and then it is not necessary. Within the scope of the evolution of humankind, a conversion, *a transformation* of energies will probably come about so that love and primal creative forces express themselves in a different way than through sexuality. It's very possible that people also enjoy life in a completely different way than through sexuality.[35] He/she who doesn't feel like this form of exchange doesn't have to bring himself/herself "into question"; look at and follow the signals which your Living Self-Core sends you, makes you feel, and trust in this. By this, the human being needs to keep following his own Nature and stay faithful to what his Living Self makes him feel.

---

[35] Also read the texts about sexual impotency and frigidity in *The Key to Self-Liberation.*

When sex becomes an addiction,[36] this represents the human being who is overflowing with creative forces and wants to allow himself to be born, "to be" more and more in matter, and intensely longs to develop himself, in autonomy and self-assuredness, not in dependence (and as a result, addiction) to "the" sexual act. He will make use of all his inherent energies in order to reach a higher and more powerful level inside himself; he will need to become "master" over his life, over himself; he will not adore anything or anyone outside himself, but will give shape to his inner heart and to his great, wonderful "I." Then, in this self-acknowledgement he will no longer want to "fill" himself with others, no longer want to fill his feeling of emptiness with the other person. He now fulfills himself, he finds himself, and in this condition of self-fulfillment and love for himself, he can, without being addicted, come to a physically tender and/or sexual relationship with someone else. Every human being needs to determine for himself or herself whether or not he/she wants to experience sexuality. It is quite possible that "sexuality" belongs to a transitional phase in humanity.

AIDS is, among other things, a signal for humanity to not just lose one's "I" in another person, in amorousness or in instinctive sexual experiences. Life asks that we allow these primal forces in us to flow from the HEART under the guidance of LOVE, whether this be in creativity or in expressing love. And as long as we just "allow ourselves to be lived" by uncontrolled urges and passions, we follow the track which completely runs away from "life." Therefore: guide yourself to your own Heart and then, as master over your own life, do what you feel you have to do. You as a completeness, experience that which is most beautiful in yourself, because of yourself, and either can or not, in physical form, bring this into expression with another person. It's this Love that counts, and whether it is between two men, two women, or between a man and a woman that doesn't matter. We should not forget here that EVERY human being carries IN himself the female and male aspect. TRUE LOVE, that's what it's about; and for those who wish so, sex can be part of this, but it is not a must. Everything is in evolution.

It's so important that someone who doesn't want sex, not do it; even not, for instance, just to please the other person, because then he/she lies to him/herself, and this will take its toll sooner or later — for instance he/she then unconsciously will attract the signal "bladder infection" or "fungal infection," etc.[37]

---

[36] Read more about sexual addiction in The Key to Self-Liberation.
[37] Read more about these illnesses in The Key to Self-Liberation.

A Sham Life Promotes Illness and Death
About Power and Manipulation

When a human being consciously or unconsciously develops and forms his or her body in order to gain "power" over another human being (through attraction, seduction, etc.) then this implies a movement of drawing in, like that of a vacuum cleaner. This is the image of dark death, which wants to get the other person in its grip, swallow him, and drag him to a deep dark hole. The story of the spider and its web, the fly is being eaten up. Men who are being dragged along in this way by the behavior, and certain physical manipulations of certain women, have to come to the realization that they allow themselves to be persuaded by "death"; that they attract this situation in order to finally "see through" sham and Death, in order to ultimately break with it and choose in favor of life, of love. Power and Seduction have NOTHING to do with love and life. The same goes for the tough guy or the "charming," unctuous man who tries to impress a woman as if he were a movie actor. Every man / woman does well to realize this. Do you still behave as a being who dresses, acts, applies certain plastic surgery (e.g., silicone implants, liposuction) or shapes your body through diet in order to develop attractive powers? In order to have more *power* over the other person because you answer more to the current norms of beauty? Know, then, that you *play along with death* and that actually this is just *outward appearance and ugliness.* Therefore, become who you really are, dress yourself in clothes that you like (that your *real* Self likes), that are comfortable on you, in colors you like, but never do something "to enchant," "to charm" someone else, to be regarded as "elegant," or "tough" or to look "cool," because then you use your self as an empty Vacuum cleaner, *then you weave a Web like a Spider in order to catch a fly. But whoever digs a pit for someone else will ultimately fall into it himself. This power-game only lasts for a certain time, and it ends in illness, decline, and death.* Why? Because this whole game is built on death and not on the basis of life — on taking and seizing and not on giving. He who sows death, ultimately kills himself.

In all parts of the world there are prevailing fashion trends or traditions and habits concerning how to be regarded "attractive": this is about SHAM, not about real beauty. Because true beauty originates in the

Heart and flows along with the truth. Truth is Life, is *giving* in love. All of the World of Appearances will sooner or later fall apart; at this moment it is true that individuals and small groups of people are already being confronted with this: *that the game of power, attraction, and suction can give brief pleasure, but it is followed by hell and decay and misery and ultimately death.* And that this kind of pleasure is NOTHING compared with TRUE ENJOYMENT . . . there, where two people let true Love reign and give to each other (also physically), without any particle of drawing in, seduction, swallowing up, addiction, false "beauty," sham forms.

It happens that people who, by birth, already have the conviction that they want to have power over others have sold their souls to the devil, so to speak, and, be it unconsciously, form a body, a face, etc., that perfectly answers to the prevailing beauty-ideal in the region in which they are born. As it is their desire to be adored and have power over others, they cultivate a body that gives them this power in a state of Sham Beauty. But their soul-core, their heart, their love-kernel, is "absent." And to those who are tuned in to true life, these masks are hideous, reeking of death; one "looks through" the game of the representatives of Lies and Death. These "people," then, are being adored by those who are also attuned to these false beauty ideals, who also allow themselves to be dragged along by the current norms of beauty. But this tale always has a fatal ending, because it is built on lies and death. Certain people act "cool," others constantly smile engagingly and "sweetly"; they entice like the Lorelei or like a fragile fairy. All life-force, all honesty, has disappeared from them; we only see a mask, a sham form. The distorted human being; the weak Eve's image, the tough Adam's image. Both types have strayed off the path called Life and Love and are holding each other in a whirlpool that pulls them down to the deep, to death.

Don't allow yourself to be led to the land of death.
Choose to truly live, in genuineness.

Being "nice and sweet" . . .
represents something else than LOVE

Being nice and sweet, "the smile," etc. is frequently a mask, a camouflage, because often there is no warm and happy heart, no real joy present. Or, if we are talking about people in a male form, with charm, charisma, or as tough, indomitable supermen. . . . There are so many forms, so many sham images — and their heart is cold or absent. Tests of the Living Self: how well do you see through "the devilish aspect" in yourself, in others? Are your endearing smile, your enticing eyes, your posture, the way in which you use your voice, like a trap in order to please the other person? This is not Love; it has nothing to do with true life.

How well are you connected with your heart, with real beauty, with honesty and authenticity . . . or do you, too, lie to life, doing your utmost to shape your body the way it has to be in order "to catch" others in your web? Then, you play with death. Do you constantly smile sweetly, automatically, like a puppet, or do you show yourself tough and strong, forever shaping your body in a "seductive" way? Then, you are an accomplice of Death, and your life will end sooner or later in "hell" (here on earth). However, if your "Laugh" is an honest expression of your Heart, then everything is okay.

So: choose the path of Life, of Giving, of Love, of Truth, of authentic Beauty: BECOME WHO YOU REALLY ARE. Live from within, not according to the eyes of others — then you will reach love and harmony with yourself, and only then can you Enjoy the Utmost in soul and body, meeting the Highest Form of Happiness in yourself or in a relationship. Because, as long as you kept roaming on the path of power and seduction, you could not — and can never — experience that high level of enjoyment, that higher happiness which grows endlessly. You then just kept stagnating in a kind of intoxication or pleasure, which doesn't reflect one billionth of the enjoyment of an exchange with a partner that grows from the root of Love.

You just kept roaming in a phase in which one gratification and one desire was immediately followed by the next . . . an endless "filling" with something that would never be able to offer you true happiness and full enjoyment. So, if you still discover in yourself something of this power system, or discover it in people you become infatuated with, know then that this world of Power and Appearances ultimately will completely destroy itself. Grow in LOVE, in AUTHENTICITY, in pureness and originality. In this honesty with himself every human being is good the way he is and this truth . . . brings Happiness.

The Cult of Looks and Appearances, or:
the schizoid dissociation in society,
within the human being himself

Dissociated? Split? In most societies one has come to see the form and the physical appearance of the human being separate from his content, his "vibrational nature." One lives "toward the mirror"; one no longer feels connected to one's inner worth. One gets estranged from oneself. This brings about diseases, be it more mental or rather physically perceptible affections.

Another consequence of this "dissociation" is that one has come to create "norms" regarding purely the outer "image." A PLUMP or THIN body, TALL or SMALL, being born with two noses, without auricles, with one leg, as a hermaphrodite, with many colored spots on one's skin, etc. — in the eyes of Life, all this is of no importance — it is all BEAUTIFUL and HEALTHY, as long as the Human Being manifests, through these physical characteristics, his True Inner Nature, in Love. Love yourself the way you *are*.

In a society where only slimness is considered "beautiful" and "healthy," there is an urge for power that wants to suppress the true, primordial, round, feminine aspect (just like the earth is round), to make it subordinate to the structurally more bony, colder, rigid masculine image. It seems that fashion designers (and those who slavishly wear these designs) totally want to suppress in themselves, and in others, the primordial, round femininity and the corresponding Forces, Potentials, Talents and Emotional Wealth (be it unconsciously — this is no reproach).[38] A deep primal anxiety lies hidden under this, only to be solved by fully integrating into oneself the true, original, feminine aspect of life. Only then, Life will open up and blossom in the human being; then, true happiness can enter and anxieties will disappear.

Flesh and fat[39] in themselves are not ugly. Flesh and fat are, in the first place, symbolic of power and energy. There's nothing wrong with a "healthy" belly[40] — which symbolizes the laugh of life, a rich Content.

---

[38] Situation at the end of the 20th century and the beginning of the 21st century.

[39] In *The Key to Self-Liberation — Encyclopedia of Psychosomatics,* the symbolic meanings of fat, muscles, and the belly are discussed.

[40] In *The Key to Self-Liberation — Encyclopedia of Psychosomatics,* the symbolic meaning of the belly is explained. This goes for people who feel good in their skin, which can then be confirmed by healthy blood test results, etc.

But in Western and other societies — when instinctive greediness and sexual organs are of prime interest, and love, the fully rounded giving, has been trampled upon — only "sex points" and "suction hollows" are allowed to exist: in order to pull in, in order to pin themselves into others . . . in order to fill their own "chilly emptiness." Bulging organs, tight clothes, but especially no belly . . . because that doesn't belong in the world of desires, of pulling in and seizing. The diet industry and sex exploitation are afraid that . . . Love might rise above Sex and Money.[41] In addition, they probably don't know that physical enjoyment only gives a real feeling of Fullness when experienced out of Love, not out of seduction, "suction" or addiction.

"Dead flesh" is the body of the person who artificially keeps himself / herself skinny (because he / she "thinks" himself / herself "too fat"). Through a strict diet, through operations (for instance, liposuction) or through inner manipulation — all of which comes down to use of power — one molds the body: it is power flesh. Of course, the same goes for the person who thinks himself / herself too skinny (here or there) and wants to "thicken" himself / herself in an artificial way.

"Living flesh," a living body, is that body which is honestly shaped from within by the person who thankfully eats — in a balanced way — what he is in the mood for[42] and doesn't "mold" his body in order to please or "catch" someone else; this human being lives in love, his body is love, is healthy, is true beauty, stout or thin, small or tall.

The greater part of humanity has strayed from heart and content. The human being clings to outer appearances — to "What do I look like?" — to something to grasp hold of outside himself. He doesn't believe in his inner divine power, in his ability to autonomously make himself happy in a self-aware way. He allows his life to be dependent on whether or not "he possesses" — perhaps this might be about material possessions, but it can just as well be about such and such a body, or this or that "partner" he has an eye on. The ideal of slenderness has, in the 20th century, become very fashionable in many parts of the world: everyone should be "skinny." One fools oneself thinking that this is the only healthy way of being: it's absurd. The ideal weight exists, yes, but it's different for every person. THE INNER NATURE

---

[41] ironically meant

[42] On condition that he "live according to Life." Read more about this elsewhere in this book. Exceptions are diabetes, alcoholism, food allergies, and other medical conditions that require dietary restrictions.

Christiane Beerlandt®, Life Philosophy – © Beerlandt Publications, Lierde, Belgium

OF A HUMAN BEING WISHES TO PLACE ITSELF IN A MATERIAL COUNTERPART. *If you are thin by nature, because of your inner character, then your nature wants to place itself in a thin body. If you are naturally round and robust, then your nature wants to place itself in a powerful, plump body.* And this doesn't mean that you are ill.

Be convinced that the outline of your body goes together with power and mobility. No matter whether you are thin or plump, live in joy, according to your true nature; live in harmony with Life, with Being. Don't dwell in spheres of "wanting to possess or acquire (this or that person, thing, goal)." Don't at all allow yourself to be fooled by the Cult of looks and appearances, which has lost every element of truth. Don't allow yourself to be fooled by drug industries and doctrines of dieting-to-lose-weight that want to make you believe that you are inevitably unhealthy if you are plump. Feel the truth yourself, uninfluenced by indoctrinations.

"Yes, but I can't walk up three flight of stairs," sighs a man. Why should this man walk up three flight of stairs if he feels it's not in his constitution? *Nor does an elephant do what a chimpanzee swinging on lianas does.* Nor does a tortoise do what a hare does. A farmer's horse is a farmer's horse, and a race horse is a race horse; we cannot compare them with each other. Don't ask a race horse to pull a heavy cart; don't ask a farmer's horse to run lots of laps. Fat in itself need not be unhealthy. (Read about this in *The Key to Self-Liberation*.) Fat definitely has its function: it's a wealth of energy, warming, and holds substances inside which, when needed, will be released in the body. *It matters that you organize your life in such a way that your actions, your movements, etc., are in harmony with your true nature. Don't force anything.* And if you live according to the conviction that you are good the way you are — unique as "you," in your body, chubby or thin — then you will attract an environment and life circumstances which, in a beneficial way, are in line with your nature. *Therefore, do the movements that suit your true nature.*

In the research that has been done into osteoporosis,[43] it has been seen that this condition occurs much less in robust women than in slender women — meaning those slender women who "artificially" keep themselves slender while their inner constitution intends them to be robust. The result is all kinds of bone fractures and hip replace-

---

[43] Read more about osteoporosis in *The Key to Self-Liberation*.

ments, etc. What matters is to be YOURSELF and become yourself, believe in your inner power . . . no matter if you are thin or plump. Your ORGANS and your complete bone structure will accommodate themselves in a way that is necessary for carrying YOUR highly unique body. We have seen many examples of stout, healthy people, more than 95 years old — healthy, because they listened to their spontaneous food likes and dislikes, and therefore needed this food in order to keep a balance between the body and the spirit. They didn't fool themselves into believing that being plump was automatically unhealthy. They felt and knew that having a full, rounded body shape can go hand in hand with power and mobility — as long as one is inwardly *convinced* of it. And PROVIDED THAT one lives "according to Life" and puts into practice what the language of one's preferred food products asks.[44] In a balanced way, one stops eating when one feels that it is good to do so: "I've had enough." This is different for everyone.

In certain countries (e.g., parts of Africa) one sees that only plumpness and roundness are considered beautiful and healthy. While writing the present book, health professionals working in these regions told me that many local women administered themselves corticoids in order to become "extra thick" so that a man would find them desirable and beautiful. Here, the opposite of the Western model prevails. Both cults-of-looks-and-appearances with their desires are equally absurd and unhealthy. This set of tricks with all kinds of means to slim down or inflate would better disappear.

Most people don't honestly place themselves in matter anymore — not only because they want to answer to the prevailing external norms ("I want to be considered beautiful and perhaps be adored, to have power"), but also because the medical world is convinced that more rotund people are necessarily unhealthy, and that being thin is healthy. (As said before, this is not the case in all parts of the world.) In practice we have seen so many people who are healthy and plump, at ninety, a hundred, or older. One needs to take into account that statistics can never prove anything really objectively because they are influenced energetically by the convictions of the researchers-statisticians, who themselves are part of a society system with its paradigms, thought patterns, established convictions, fashion trends and norms.

---

[44] Read more about this subject in the book *The Horn of Plenty* (not yet published in English at the time of the publication of the present book).

Furthermore, many plump, robust people only begin to feel pain in their hearts within a Western society where they are treated disrespectfully, reproached, condemned for their physical appearance. They then anxiously turn to pills, for instance, follow strict diets, etc. In sum, *they don't dare be themselves anymore, and they become sad* (sometimes, as a result, they may develop type 2 diabetes, for instance[45]). They no longer believe in their authentic beauty, in their power and mobility. Ultimately, they fall ill. An *ideal weight* by itself — with all sorts of charts of height, weight, calories, etc. — *does not exist*. The human being with his "rationality" has strayed far away from wisdom and clear insight. He wants to change a round orange into a thin soy sprout and the other way round, and doesn't at all listen anymore to the language of his inner nature. *Content and Form in Balance, in Harmony with each other* — *that* means health. So, it cannot be otherwise than there are healthy plump and healthy slim people walking around on this earth. Every human being is unique.

It's even *necessary* that spirit and content, consciousness and matter remain in Harmony and Balance: certain people with a strong energy field, formidable creative powers, emotional riches, a wealth of talents and abilities, require sometimes a robust, stout body as a counterpart. Put these people on a very harsh diet, and they could fall ill. A large number of young people even die from anorexia nervosa.

Anorexia nervosa represents the behavior, carried to extremes, of a person who wants power via a "thin" appearance, who wants to be considered beautiful by others (at least within a society where thinness is the standard or the ideal) — instead of *offering herself or himself love* and allowing herself or himself to grow and expand the way nature in her or him wants it. One wants to please others, to attract all the *attention,* and ultimately one receives visitors in the hospital, lonely, because eventually the "previous friends" also fall away. In this way, a life filled with sucking in attention and power ultimately ends very sadly.

Therefore, it cannot be repeated too many times to everyone: become who you really are; lovingly give yourself the full attention. Don't compare yourself with anyone; don't listen to the *herd-mentality* of a superficial sham-world. Follow only YOUR DEEP LIFE CORE, your

---

[45] The psycho-emotional origins of Diabetes are discussed in *The Key to Self-Liberation*. Addressing these psychological undercurrents does not at all exclude the need for thorough medical follow-up, dietary measures, etc.

HEART, the voice of truth very deep inside you. Allow your body to be an honest manifestation, powerful and healthy, of who you *really* are. This truth means health, joy, and beauty.

Food and Health
Listen to your Body,
listen to your Living Self

Live in thankfulness, enjoy in thankfulness, eat delicious food in thankfulness. Not instinctively but consciously, in the fullness of love.
When you are hungry, eat what you are in the mood for at that moment (without going to extremes, of course), *because your soul-core indicates to you via this taste what food product you now need most, according to soul, psyche, and body.*

Here, an **EXCEPTION** needs to be made for illnesses such as diabetes, alcoholism and other addictions, food allergies or intolerances, heart and blood vessel conditions, high blood pressure, certain metabolic disorders, etc. In these cases, the underlying psychological issue should be solved first and, of course, dietary measures have to be observed when medically necessary.

If you are in the mood for an apple, then don't eat a pear. If you feel like having chocolate, then eat it.[46] Do you not like raw vegetables, nor whole wheat bread, but do you prefer white bread and steamed red cabbage? Well then eat that. Do you like potatoes? Then they are healthy for you, provided that the abovementioned exceptions are taken into account.

Still, there are also other **CONDITIONS** attached to this. *Live "according to truth" in your daily existence. Therefore, also listen to the "language" of the food product(s) that you like to eat; bring into practice what this food asks you to do.*[47] These conditions and the issue of "Living according to Life" are also discussed elsewhere in the present book.

---

[46] Except in case of certain illnesses, as already underlined.
[47] Read about this in *The Horn of Plenty* (not yet published in English at the time of the publication of the present book).

Do you feel bad after consuming certain food products? Then don't eat them. Do you feel bad in your skin? Then make the necessary changes in your life, from out of your heart; only YOU, YOURSELF, can feel and know what these changes are. Do you feel that you need more movement? Then don't keep sitting for hours in front of your computer or TV! Etc.

The human being has lost trust in this natural taste. When you eat what you like — provided that in everyday life, you **really** put into practice the symbolic language of the food you eat, and that you *"live according to Life"* — then you will grow toward the bodily shape and body weight that is ideal for you. Then your body is the ideal reflection of your specific vibration field — and that's good. That's ideal in order to achieve or keep an optimal state of health. And, whether you should lose weight or gain weight, you can only find out which shape *really* belongs to your Content — and renders your specific Frequency of Being — if you follow your natural, spontaneous likings . . . on the condition, however, that you don't force yourself, that you always "live according to Life," not according to Appearances, not according to the conviction "that you are not allowed to be who you *are.*"

Also, you learn to understand the "signals" you encounter on your life path.[48] Then you don't go to extremes but feel calm and in balance. It speaks for itself that someone who doesn't live according to Life — and for instance sits around entire days — ultimately brings himself into a state of sleep, creating an immobile body, and his organs will become ill. But the opposite is also true: the person who forces himself every day to do sports and run — while he inwardly feels that he's going too far and his inner self says "stop" — might well make himself ill. Therefore, follow your sense of truth and put into practice that which your Living Self-Core asks you.

Very important: every food product you long for — that is which your body and your psyche have a need for because you unconsciously want to bring yourself into greater harmony and health — *every food product speaks "a language" which you have to listen to.* For instance: someone who longs for a tomato has a need to bring his joy outward in an extroverted way, not hiding himself in an introverted way. As, for

---

[48] The underlying meanings of occurrences as signposts on your life's path are discussed in *The Signal Book* (not yet published in English at the time of the publication of the present book).

instance, milk chocolate says: deal with yourself in a soft, warm, flexible, loving feminine way, don't dig in your heels, etc., etc. . . .

If you do NOT listen to the language of Life — if you don't put into practice that which the food product you long for asks you to do — then you could fall ill. Therefore, you cannot just eat everything without any problem.

In the book *The Horn of Plenty,*[49] the meaning of several hundred food products is explained, called up "according to truth." *In this way, you can learn to understand yourself better according to what you like to eat, and become more conscious of what Life in you asks of you.*

Only that person becomes ill who doesn't live according to life, doesn't love himself, disregards the signals on his life path, doesn't live in joy, in thankfulness for his Being. For instance, someone can be convinced "that he is immobile, that he is weak or limp." As a result of this conviction, certain thin people, for instance, will develop an illness that prevents them from standing on their legs, while certain thick people won't be able to get out of their chair anymore. Both examples have by themselves nothing to do with being thin or thick. It's about the specific conviction one carries within . . . and according to which one lives. As pointed out before, one need not feel guilty about this. Always be understanding toward yourself and your evolution process. Bring about changes in your life pattern when it is necessary.

Therefore, we can see two people who both weigh 100 lbs. and one of them will be as healthy and mobile as a hare, whereas the other's legs give way under him; in the same way we can see two people both weighing more than 200 lbs. the one going through life vigorously, dynamically and very solidly, while the other one sorrows, droops in a chair, considers himself sick, and can no longer stand on his legs.

Arrive at the truth, at true beauty, at Living Power — because very often the human being doesn't even know anymore what that is. *Life itself never fixates on the external form but always grows from within.*

When you really do, and put into practice, that which the food product you fancy "asks" of you, then you live "according to

---

[49] This book hasn't yet been published in English at the time of the publication of the present book

Life" or "according to truth," at least with regard to this point or aspect.

For instance, having an appetite for **strawberries** asks you, among other things, to arrive at a healthy awareness of your personal worth, to assertively draw your boundaries in relation to others when they want to penetrate too much into your personal domain. In this way, different aspects can need your attention. Put into practice that which your spontaneous food preferences ask of you. This will only benefit your personal development and your physical health.

It speaks for itself that someone who already has "diabetes"[50] should not right away start eating loads of sugar, but first needs to solve the psycho-emotional origins of diabetes in himself in a very fundamental way. Only then, if the pancreas begins to function better and better under the influence of the psychological changes being applied, one can try very cautiously to gradually authorize more food products containing sugar in the daily diet again. We have had the joy to see this course of events with certain people who cured themselves of diabetes. Of course, all of this always needs to be done in consultation with, and under supervision of, an experienced and qualified physician or medical team.

Eating when you are hungry is healthy.[51] Don't confuse eating a lot with "gluttony" or bulimia. Gluttony is precisely the result of the human being constantly putting the breaks on eating normally, because he is convinced that "eating the food he feels a need for" would be bad for him (unhealthy, or not good for "the figure"),[52] and because he wants to please others with a physical appearance that corresponds to the received norms of society. In other words, he denies himself a certain food product or permission to eat a healthy quantity of it. Because of this, his Life-Core will sooner or later force this human being to take in what he refuses to give to himself. Then, at a certain moment, he can do nothing but suddenly throw himself upon the Food, emptying the refrigerator. In this way, he falls into extremes. For instance, he denies himself a delicious little piece of chocolate, again and again; as

---

[50] Diabetes is discussed at length in *The Key to Self-Liberation — Encyclopedia of Psychosomatics*. More information about sugar and sweets can be found in *The Horn of Plenty* (not yet published in English at the time of the publication of the present book).
[51] Except when certain foods are not allowed for medical reasons.
[52] Here, the person doesn't consider that it is healthy to listen to his spontaneous food preferences on the condition that he put into practice that which the food product he fancies asks him to do. Read more about this in the book *The Horn of Plenty,* which hasn't yet been published in English at the time of the publication of the present book.

time goes by, the result may be that he feels like gobbling up tons of it at once. Of course, this is an unhealthy situation.

If this person also has a "feeling of guilt" while eating certain food products, then, so to speak, the brain "refuses" to send a signal of satisfaction. The result is that gluttony is stimulated even more. That's why *the* cure for gluttony or bulimia says: eat what you are in the mood for, *without* feelings of guilt.[53] Then, with moderation, you just take in what your body and psyche need. Eating has in itself nothing to do with "greediness," but with maintaining or promoting health and harmony. Once again, **on the condition that you "live according to Life**."

Certain people can eat much and always remain thin. Others eat the same amount of the same food and are plump. Because the form is the expression of a very specific nature. Being chubby or (honestly) thin never has to be a problem — the conditions to be put on this have been discussed above. Don't fixate on the external form but live from out of your heart.

Healthily thin or healthily plump, become who you are. Live according to the conviction that you are Powerful, Mobile, and Healthy. Live "according to Life" and do what the language of the foodstuff asks you to do.[54] Disregard the Cult of Looks and Appearances. Arrive at pure Self-Love, Self-Appreciation, and consume the food in gratitude. Do the movements that suit your nature.

Learning to *feel,* to sense how much and what to eat; this is different for each human being

Almost no one on our Earth lives a hundred percent "according to Life." Therefore — no matter how well you put into practice what the food you eat asks from you — feel, sense when you've eaten enough.

It's important to get to know yourself better and better. Just think of the symbolic meanings of salt and sugar. So, "**with moderation**" is

[53] Except when one is already "ill" and caution is advised: for instance, in diabetes patients.
[54] Read more about this in the book *The Horn of Plenty,* which hasn't yet been published in English at the time of the publication of the present book.

Christiane Beerlandt®, Life Philosophy – © Beerlandt Publications, Lierde, Belgium

mostly the motto. A **balanced** eating pattern — this is different for each human being.

This "ability to feel" is very important for your well-being. For instance, it can occur that at body and soul level you have a great need for drinking much water or eating many avocadoes, etc., and that you feel deep inside: "This is like a medicine for me now." Then don't say "no." But in general, the human being feels best when he doesn't gorge himself.

Enjoying in Thankfulness

Finally, why would we live from "light" only? Why would we say "no" to the delicious foods that life offers us as a Horn of Plenty? Let's enjoy thankfully — knowing that, should it ever be good for the human being and humankind *not* to eat anymore, then this would happen as a matter of course, in a completely natural way, without difficulty or effort. Famine in certain parts of the world won't be solved fundamentally by "fasting" or living from "light" in the so-called "rich" countries; it requires total reconsideration. One needs to become aware of "how life can work quite differently." Fundamental causes and solutions need to be looked at in order that changes can be made.

•

Heredity?
The Genes: a Dynamic Entity

A human being is not "just" haphazardly born somewhere. He is born to those parents and in that place in the world where his Living Self-Core directs him. And then he attracts — *be it unconsciously* — a genetic heritage, which he needs in order to work on himself, as a reflection of that which symbolizes him. But, *there's no question of things being "predetermined"!* Unconsciously, you have brought yourself here, within this family, in order to show yourself a "mirror" of certain things you want to solve in yourself so that you can make yourself into a happier human being. There's a kind of genetic pattern — **a genetic disposition** — in every human being, but he remains free to develop these patterns in whichever direction.

Genes, cells, etc. are not "static," predetermined elements. They are in constant agreement with the psycho-emotional movements in the human being, with his underlying conviction-field that evolves. And, therefore: genes are also in movement, susceptible to evolution and changes.

The conscious mind or unconscious convictions influence the evolution of the genetic system.

Say that you, as a young man, are born with a "father" who has a heart condition, and you, too, have it . . . and someone says "that you, too, will die when you are forty, just like your father, because it's hereditary." You don't have to believe any of this; you look up what the "heart"[55] is symbolic of, and you will see that the heart among other things asks for absolute love for yourself, joy for your existence, and especially no sham, no false appearances, no hardness, no image-striving, no exaggerated thinking with regard to feeling. The heart wants you to live in a gentle, honest, sensitive way toward yourself. Imagine the young man has seen his father living in a hard way, an image-striving way, and decides to take another path — what happens then? Together with his own psycho-emotional changes, the genes, the cells, also undergo a "transfiguration" — yes, simultaneously; matter, the material, the physical, is constantly being influenced by the spirit, by consciousness, by thoughts, emotions, expectations, convictions (conscious or unconscious).

So, thanks to insight and the bringing about of changes in the psycho-emotional field, genetic patterns alter[56] . . . and the son, in our example, never has to develop a heart condition and die early. On the contrary, the hereditary heart condition can redirect itself; the heart can regenerate and begin to experience itself — and move — in a completely different, healthier way.

There are numerous **examples** like this. Did your "mother" or your "grandmother," die of cancer, and are you, as the daughter, afraid that

---

[55] The symbolism of the heart is discussed in *The Key to Self-Liberation — Encyclopedia of Psychosomatics*.

[56] Intellectual disability takes place at another level, mostly not very "consciously" but unconsciously. It has its specific meaning for the human being himself, his environment, the society in which he lives. This is discussed more at length in *The Key to Self-Liberation — Encyclopedia of Psychosomatics*.

you will develop the same illness because of "genetic inheritance"?[57] Then, look at what cancer symbolizes.[58] Bring about changes — in other words don't live at all in the same way as your mother and grandmother did. Understand the true reason why cancer finally can develop. Thanks to the changes you bring about in your life, the genetic pattern, too, will alter, and you will never get cancer. This is the liberating message of self-healing: you can do much more than you think, much, much more! Many examples have confirmed this. So, there need be no fatalism.

Disabled persons are not necessarily sick people. For certain underlying reasons they have developed another form of functioning. This is discussed in *The Key to Self-Liberation — Encyclopedia of Psychosomatics*.

The Labyrinth and the Way Out
Death as the Last Disease to Overcome [59]

In all kinds of myths and tales, in old and new writings, profane as well as religious stories, the image of The Labyrinth, or of the "being lost" is brought to the fore. And that tells a lot about the experiences and convictions that existed in humankind and still are existing in us. The motif of the maze, of searching and (not) finding a way out. This image of The Labyrinth has come to be in the human being and stayed alive because he kept looking for "true Life," "true creative power," and "true Happiness" OUTSIDE himself. In the past (and still today), he has devised and walked a multitude of paths in order to find Life and Happiness outside himself, but they've all turned out to be dead-end roads. The human being carries within himself the memory of a myriad of roads that all end up in death.

Still: the Living Self within the human being wants to show him the Way Out, like the thread of Ariadne; the path to True Life, to Liberation. Indeed, many fairy tales and myths — which are, after all, a reflection

---

[57] More texts about genetic inheritance and congenital diseases can be found in *The Key to Self-Liberation — Encyclopedia of Psychosomatics*.
[58] The fundamental, psycho-emotional undercurrents of cancer are discussed in *The Key to Self-Liberation — Encyclopedia of Psychosomatics*.
[59] This is discussed at length in the book *New Days*, which hasn't yet been published in English at the time of the publication of the present book.

of that which lives deep inside humankind — also tell us how the human being ultimately finds a way out, no matter how precarious the situation he was in.

The only true way out will always be there, where the human being finds himself again, loves himself, Believes in himself and *knows,* very deep inside himself that he, himself, can build his life in freedom and happiness. That nothing or no one above or outside himself can break down and threaten his life; that he *himself* attracts all — yes all — situations in his life, consciously or unconsciously. The more conscious a human being becomes of this, the sooner he can deal with, and make an end to, the feeling of being stuck in a blind-alley maze. He will find, INSIDE himself, the thread of Ariadne and the path to Life without an end, to Freedom.

Concepts from the past such as "the fall of man" can be seen in this way: during the incarnation process — the birth of the human being in the earthly dimension — one has fallen into the wrong convictions, not (or no longer) believing in one's inner, divine powers, in one's goodness and ability to take one's life into one's own hands and building it into something wonderful — yes *"the primordial doubt."* The result is a desire to find *something to hold on to* in all kinds of powers and forces outside of oneself; a desire to fill oneself with things or people from the outside, with covetousness, anxiety and greed . . . straying away from one's own Fullness. Humankind didn't recognize its own magnificence full of love (anymore). The human being lost the contact with his Living Self-Core, with the True Life inside him.

The path to Ultimate Happiness, to eternal life without suffering and pain — yes, finally to physical immortality, which is the ultimate goal of life — this thread which leads us out of the labyrinth where humankind for so long has kept itself shackled, is the language of our own supreme Living Self, of our Inner Heart. And to show us this Way, our Living Center sends all kinds of Signals on our Path, to make CLEAR to us: THERE lies the way to liberation, THERE you go wrong, or here you go right; ALTER YOUR COURSE. We just have to follow this "thread" to the way out. This can be done by opening yourself up, by looking at and listening to that which the Signals in and around you can make clear — and by no longer doubting the good outcome.

•

Learning to "see" and "understand" Signals — without fanaticism

Signals, fortunately, are being constantly sent to us, or even better: we call them up ourselves (mostly unconsciously) from out of our deepest Life Essence; in this way it is made clear to us what Life in us wants, what is best for us. Signals can be "pleasant" or "unpleasant."[60] In any case they serve as *signposts* that show us where we are right or wrong. Next to the language of *illness* and *emotions,* which are very important signals that indicate "where we have to change our course," there are also the ordinary everyday happenings — apparently "just accidentally" happening to us, but this is not true.

When, for instance, a light bulb in the house pops, then this indeed has something to do with the material and technical side of things (the bulb was perhaps very old, etc.). But, still, you will see that this happening didn't just "accidentally" occur in *that* place, in the presence of *that* person, at *this* certain moment. It's always about a synchronicity, things that occur at the same time: on the one hand a light bulb that pops or lightning that hits, a glass that breaks, etc., and on the other hand "a happening" in the human being himself, in his psyche, his head, his total being. Why does this or that just happen NOW in a human life?

The energy that is too hard, sometimes too structurally cutting, the holding-on to old patterns and not being open to the stream of spontaneous, emotional, renewing energies: *that's* what the signal, "a light bulb pops," wants to say. It becomes a strong admonition when, during a certain period, many bulbs in the house pop. Then, no longer be hard to yourself; learn to relax; don't think in such a "hard" way anymore; don't stay tense within old structural habits; free yourself from

---

[60] However, *The Signal Book* mainly discusses "unpleasant" signals because they can be like hinge points in one's life if the "why" is understood well: a turn toward a happier life path.

old thinking patterns.[61]   Understand this "signal" of the light bulbs; change your way of life, and in this way you can, for instance, avoid heart palpitations.

No matter if it's about a flat tire, a theft, a car accident, a fire in the house — or whatever — it tells us SO MUCH about ourselves. I have seen that even the greatest skeptics — those who didn't believe anything of it — when they read the texts about the "signals" that were of relevance to them, they confirmed in astonishment that this situation as described in its psycho-emotional meaning was indeed "true" for them. I, therefore, advise the reader **to not simply believe anything, but neither just reject anything**. A healthy, sensible, thinking person first reflects, "opens" himself up to investigation, and doesn't reject things beforehand. Only afterwards does he draw his conclusion. Many people seem to be afraid of a deeper truth, of the language of Life itself which "speaks" via signals. It's a pleasant, educational path to walk, without having to become fanatical in this regard. Does something attract your attention? Are you forced to look at something — for instance, you break a glass twice in a row, or you lose your wallet? Then think about it, just reflect for a moment: why does this happen to me now? Read, if you like, the explanation for these happenings in *The Signal Book,* or try to figure it out yourself. Very often I have seen that, when someone became "aware" of **the *true* underlying reason** for "losing" an object, and was prepared to bring about the necessary changes in his life, then the lost object almost immediately was brought back or found. These are just a few examples of how wonderfully life functions, and how beautifully we can learn to understand it and guide it ourselves.

Nothing happens to you "just like that"

Occurrences, phenomena or illnesses that happen to you, are not "just" there all of a sudden; they don't come falling from the sky, nor are they being sent to you by one or another force or god. Everything in the world is energetically connected, to a greater or lesser extent. **You, yourself, attract everything in an energetic way. All happen-**

---

[61] The deeper meaning of several hundred signals is discussed in *The Signal Book.* This work hasn't yet been published in English at the time of the publication of the present book.

ings and phenomena are there as an externalization of something that happens on a deeper level: in your psyche, your emotional life, in your conviction-and-expectation pattern. In this way the human being creates his life, calls up situations himself, good and bad. Mostly, this all happens unconsciously, which is why people say "it just happened" again to me. *One simply is not aware that everything is energetically connected (under the surface of what we can observe with our senses), and that the human being constantly creates his reality according to his own expectations and psychological patterns.* If he becomes aware of this, then he will realize that things don't happen to him "just like that," then he himself will take his life in hand. He will then be able to look into himself and solve the deeper causes of certain unpleasant circumstances that are affecting him. He adjusts his course so that he doesn't have to encounter yet another (greater) Signal which makes the same thing clear to him, but with consequences that are much worse.

So, the human being, if applying what the Signals make clear to him, will ultimately encounter only joyful happenings on his path. The human being becomes *conscious;* he realizes, now, that only he can change his life, alter its course in the direction of goodness, truth, and happiness, so that nothing sad has to meet him anymore. **This, then, is one of the most deep-seated convictions that the human being has to deal with and make an end to: that he is born in order to suffer**, that it cannot be otherwise than for a human being to encounter unpleasant circumstances on his path of life, that he would not be able to take his life in his own hands and incline it toward constant Joy. If he breaks with this lie in himself and listens to the Signals on his path, then he will experience how he will see ever more clearly in life, how finally his Living Self will no longer attract any unpleasant signal. Give yourself time in this evolution. Be patient with yourself.

Fatalism will only play a part in your life as long as you believe in it. Everything has a reason for being: observe it. Don't close your eyes to the road signs, the Signals on your path. Take your life in hand and guide yourself ever further along: fatalism no longer exists.
Occurrences, illness, etc., are like Signals; always ask yourself "Why"? and then correct your course. "Why is there an electric short in my house? Why that flood, that earthquake? Why does my left foot fall asleep so often? What's the reason my bike got stolen? What's the

reason I have attracted this?"[62] In this way, if you already look at the smallest signals, you no longer have to attract the larger signals. *If, however, you refuse to listen to the message of small signals, then your Living Self will send you ever-greater signals — negative, serious happenings, illness — so that you finally will realize:* I am on the wrong path, the path that leads to suffering and death. Change your course! Look at the causes of these signals and solve them in yourself, so that you will reach one step farther on the path to more Life, more Joy. Without feelings of guilt! Every human being is in evolution.

That which happens on an individual level also happens en masse. However, it's up to the individual who lives consciously to start with himself first, in an autonomous way, so that a snowball effect can come into play in the world.

Finally, only "living" human beings attract "signals." *Therefore, when you encounter a "signal" on your path, don't be ashamed, don't feel yourself to be a failure, don't feel guilty.* Quite the contrary. When you are prepared to look at the deeper meaning of your signals, without pointing your finger at someone else, then this is *marvelous.* After all, by *an honest self-examination* you help yourself along, and therefore also humanity. *Becoming aware is an essential basic pillar for constructing a happy world.* Therefore, let us all be thankful for the signposts we meet on our path of life.

An Example to Clarify This

A middle-aged man called N. told his friend K. that he suffered from terrible BACKACHES, SHOULDER ACHES, etc.

N. ran a business by the seaside and the **heavy burdens** were beyond his strength. In the evening he told that his heart was "running wild" (see extrasystoles, arrhythmia), that he had a headache and pain in the knee.[63] He took remedies: herbs as well as conventional medicine. His symptoms improved.

---

[62] Read about this in *The Signal Book*. This work hasn't yet been published in English at the time of the publication of the present book.
[63] The psycho-emotional origins of these ailments are discussed in *The Key to Self-Liberation.*

He had a craving for **milk chocolate**; the chocolate did him good at the level of his soul and body. At that moment, he did not yet realize that it worked as a "medicine"[64] in order to help him sustain unbearable burdens (his too heavy workload).

> Milk chocolate stands for receptiveness. It stimulates the human being to take in gentle energies that are being supplied. The inner, mild flows, born in the depths of the Self, work their way upward; they ask the human being to offer them a Gate, an Opening of re-ceptiveness through which the life forces full of love may enter — in order to finally fill his entire being with love, gentleness, suppleness, flexibility, life-warmth, leniency, motherly understanding.
>
> . . .
>
> Milk chocolate asks you to "bend the knee" and yield, there where you have been maintaining a "stiff position" for too long (to your own detriment!) "Don't keep your doors closed any longer. Let it all flow in from deep down your diaphragm, your inner Life-Source. Allow this smooth, mildly warm flood full of love to stream through your entire body and to purge you of every war, tension, struggle, re-sistance to life. Become one with this gentleness, with this love and, especially, DON'T RESIST!" That's what chocolate says.
>
> Excerpt from *The Horn of Plenty —*
> *Psychological, Symbolic Language of Foodstuffs*[65]

The sixth week of the busy summer months he drove tired to his home. At a traffic circle, his car collided with another vehicle; the car window shattered into a thousand pieces. The doctor examined him; nothing serious, but he did have terrible pain in the neck, the back, the shoul-ders, the knees . . . .

He was very frightened by the incident and talked about it with his friend K., who pointed out to him the symbolism of a **car accident** as explained in *The Signal Book:*

> You KEEP HOLD of things or people — as if you are carrying a heavy rucksack on your shoulders — and you refuse to let go of that

---

[64] Please note that there are conditions attached to this. See elsewhere in this book.
[65] This work has not yet been published in English at the time of the publication of the present book.

which blocks your free path of life. Will you finally make a true move, or not? A mass of energies are stored. But you DON'T DO anything really creative with them — or maybe you direct them in a totally wrong way: by living in desire, in possessiveness, in occupations that are too superficial. Meanwhile, your inner core calls for a TRUE BIRTH OF YOUR "I," IN ALL ITS MAGNIFICENCE. So, you deviate from the straight path. Do you attach importance to false values? Have you been trying to keep things as close to you as possible, to hold on to what you have — instead of allowing all your powers, talents, content . . . to flow through, thus allowing innovation? You seem to be hesitating in which direction you would go with your content, with your supplies. But you do keep everything with you, for yourself.

. . .

You are bursting with potential . . . but you don't launch yourself. Energies are being held back; you bloat your rucksack but you don't unload. True Mars-powers do not straightly come out; they look for a discharge via a detour. You are not entirely on the right track. You somehow keep yourself away from the true life path (where, after all, your happiness lies). "I can't . . . ," these are the worlds that are possibly sounding in your soul; a feeling of powerlessness, of "life-impotency." It is important to understand that you don't need to KEEP anything, that you don't need to hold on to anything. It's a good thing if you give yourself up to life. You may let everything flow out of you; you share and give, with a generous heart, to yourself and to people whom you cherish.

Arrive at true creation; don't confine yourself to a narrow field. Don't keep it all in, don't bottle it up, don't heap up your content like this; instead, relax and TRUST that way through, that free passage. Grant yourself a free discharge.

. . .

You have DEVIATED from the true path of life; you are off on a SIDETRACK in life and will have to bring yourself back to the straight path: there where you can let yourself be who you really are from within, in freedom and joy — without having to concern yourself too much with the practical, material, external, empty side of things. As long as you block LIFE in the fullest sense of the word — as long as you AMASS, HOLD ON TO things, and FIX your ATTENTION on things that actually have nothing to do with life — you will "collide" with life, with the living self-core in you which asks nothing more than that you would give yourself the freedom and happiness.

Excerpt from *The Signal Book* [66]

He, N., who had never fancied **milk**, suddenly felt like having large quantities of milk. He didn't understand a thing about it.

. . . the human being who has decided not to let himself go but to *implement the new*. He who longs for "getting started," for his "I" to get into its stride, **for a "beginning" movement** which goes further, always further . . . . He stands at the starting line to set off shortly. Virgin grounds have to be explored. He has an optimistic perspective on it; he is full of hope and courage. It is all still so new, and he longs for becoming the Writer of his Life Story himself. He himself will begin to fill in his blank book — or he will start to write a new book.

The atmosphere of Milk is one of OPENNESS, a feeling of openness, an open outlook — the typical happy and free feeling before one can start the New (every day again).

The feeling of **a New Start**; everything has to, or can, begin now — or start all over. You feel: "I am at the beginning; I can still do so much, go so far." An unreachable Horizon; a Path that will never be finished. The human being is ready to go. The milk atmosphere opens up the brain, the mind, the heart, the view, the senses. One looks far, very far ahead. Courage, force, daring, freshness, an available store . . . .

Excerpt from *The Horn of Plenty — Psychological, Symbolic Language of Foodstuffs:* the chapter about milk [67]

Also quoted below are two texts from *The Key to Self-Liberation — Encyclopedia of Psychosomatics:* the text about heart arrhythmia (abnormality of the rhythm of the heart) and the one about extrasystoles (the heart skips a beat), which began to bother him more and more.

---

[66] This work has not yet been published in English at the time of the publication of the present book.
[67] This work has not yet been published in English at the time of the publication of the present book.

Fundamental, psycho-emotional origin of and solution to **heart ar-rhythmia**, in general:

Fundamental Origin

Unsure, indecisive, seeking in several directions at once. . . . Confused thoughts; you get many contradictory impressions: you are a slave of them, cannot handle them all. You don't follow a straight line, don't take a clear stand. You cannot say farewell to something or someone even though the facts indicate you should let go and go on. You think and fret in a vicious circle because you don't have enough faith in your Self, in your intuition. You are stuck, as it were, with your head in something, in someone. You'd like to tear yourself loose, but your feeling of dependence and your lack of self-worth, the under-appreciation of yourself, cause you to suppress yourself: your feelings, your longings, your autonomous self-realization.

You cannot bet on two horses at the same time: first and foremost, you have to make choices that are for your own good and for the sake of your health. This dilemma — yourself or your surroundings? — is the consequence of unbalanced seeking for yourself. You want to do good for others, but also for yourself; you might do too much for others so that they would accept you, so that they would like you. Because of this, you are holding yourself back and don't live resolutely in *one* direction. You are being pulled in two directions; this tension is becoming too heavy a burden for you.

It could equally as well be a dilemma of having to choose something involving your job, your relations — a nervous, insecure quest: yes / no / yes . . . jerking and jolting along.

Fundamental Solution

Stay close to your feelings, your intuition, and don't fill your head with confused thoughts. Allow all emotions to flow freely, don't bottle them up, fret no longer, let go of that which causes inner collisions. Quietly take time for yourself; don't let yourself be rushed by others. Follow your true nature: trust this and go on your way, imperturbably, without letting yourself be deviated by the opinions of others. Say farewell to certain views, or bring about changes in oppressive situations. First of all, achieve peaceful harmony in yourself and trust that your environment will be a reflection of this. Make a choice, determine your direction, and go onward in a steady rhythm. Trustingly follow the signals that life sends you on your path, and everything will work out fine.

Excerpt from *The Key to Self-Liberation*

Fundamental, psycho-emotional origin of and solution to **extrasystoles** ("Your heart skips a beat"):

Your legs, *tired* and walked on until they are bowed, as it were, dead-tired. You finally don't know anymore how far you have gone already, *for how long you have been persevering in this direction* (literally or figuratively), but one thing is definite: it has been going on for a long time! But you keep on going on and on and on, so that your legs might take on an O shape. You probably think *it all HAS TO BE that way,* just like the long distance runner or jogger who is totally convinced that this or that distance *must* be covered: *that it is supposed to be that way,* or for the sake of fitness; in the meantime one doesn't realize that one causes oneself to grow older and shrink instead of becoming healthier, but one is convinced that it *is* okay, no matter how much effort it costs!

Life itself doesn't ask for this. Why such insistent, fixed ideas? Why still live according to "oppressive laws" without questioning them? *Use YOUR INDIVIDUALITY, your highly unique thinking Ability, in order to place it all in question . . . and to see where you constantly FORCE, EXHAUST, push yourself, where you do things that are hard for you, where you absolutely keep it up and don't even question: "Is this LIFE; is this really good for me?" Then stand still . . . and think about this. See how you have forced yourself to keep on walking in a tense way for too long, have acted or thought strenuously in this or that direction, in this or that hard way.* Now take away those blinders.

Stop "following," doing what's "supposed to be done," what others, or society, norms, and rules tell you to do "because it's good for you." FOLLOW YOUR HIGHLY UNIQUE PATH in a loving, but truly creative way. After all you are not a monkey, not an imitator, not an idiot who runs in circles or does this or that every night because "someone" says that's how it's supposed to be . . . that's how it has to be . . . as if YOU are not allowed to exist as YOU! As if life asks you for strong efforts!

Time to change the rudder: you live from your inner Feeling, from your heart. It's okay for you to work and make efforts, build up thoughts, but as long as they don't hurt you, as long as they are not "pushed on you" by doctrines, habits, social norms or whatever. You do take responsibility for your existence, but you now begin to live from out of your creative "I"-thinking and your supervising brain!

Stop walking on in this way. Reconsider everything. Look at *where* you just do and follow what the rules and others and society have told you to do: realize then that LIFE doesn't ask that from you. *IN-DEPTH UNDERSTANDING is being asked; possibly seeing through certain indoctrinations which make you give importance to things of no importance.* Go back to the source inside yourself and ask yourself what's GOOD for YOU personally.

An *example:* don't live automatically or think that sport is healthy because everyone says so. Know why you need this or that food product and why your body enjoys it, no matter if it's chocolate or pears. Know that nothing is unhealthy if the signal comes from out of your deepest self, from your soul-center upwards, and tells you to take this or that. But at the same time understand the cause of your liking this or that food product, and work at it.[68] A human being is HEALTHY when he JOYFULLY experiences his own nature and does what he feels he has to do, from out of his deepest self — not because it "has to be that way" or because that's "the way it's done."

BE . . . BECOME who you *really* are! Also regarding the exterior: don't allow yourself to be fooled into believing that only skinny muscles are healthy, and fat would inevitably be unhealthy, that you have to be slim at all costs, and being heavy would automatically be bad or unhealthy. FEEL what is good and healthy for you, and also see through the cult of looks and appearances: true beauty lies in the extension of truth, not in someone who creates a body made to manipulate with power, emptied inside and filling himself with things and/or people from the outside.

No longer ACHIEVE on any level, but just be yourself: live according to the truth, from your heart, in goodness, and *SEE THROUGH* things, look for *the ESSENCE,* for *the CONTENT* of life, no longer FORCING yourself in order to GET, *to want TO HAVE* this or that. *Let go! Arrive at the vibration of BEING instead of HAVING!* And this "having" doesn't necessarily have anything to do with material

---

[68] Please note that there are important conditions attached to this. See the chapter "Food and Health" in this book.

things (although this is also possible), but it can be about *"wanting to have a certain situation" that is not there (yet)* . . . and you WANT this to come to be. *LET GO! Don't force anything; and trust. Experience the joy of your "Being."*

Stop making it so hard for yourself, stop also FILLING yourself with the things you think to be IMPORTANT but which in fact in the view of Life itself are of no importance. Listen to that gentle but resolute voice of your inner heart and follow only that path. Don't live on the SURFACE, on the outside of your being, but live and act from out of your deepest source, according to what you feel deep inside. *It's necessary to look THROUGH things,* to realize thoroughly that everything has a reason.

DON'T JUST KEEP ON WALKING ON AND ON without coming to the realization of the fact that there lies something MUCH deeper under the surface and false layers — search for that information of truth. This can be done by no longer thoughtlessly doing things the way you used to, by no longer keeping on going in a direction you used to think you were supposed to go in. Now listen to your inner ear. WHAT does your heart really want? *What* does life ask? No longer make yourself so tense. No longer fill yourself with things, but EXPERIENCE YOURSELF in your own fullness; enjoy your being. Don't just be occupied with your work, or with just what you do or achieve, but *connect yourself with your INNER CORE OF FEELING, with your heart; then FEEL how it calls for a "stop," NOT KEEPING ON RUNNING the way you are at the moment . . . in thoughts and meditations or in deeds.*

Return to your deepest source, turn deeply inward, be good and gentle with yourself. Stop "filling" yourself, and now fulfill yourself completely with the love that will flow through your total being. *For a while stop living, thinking, working, organizing at the Surface . . . and listen to the deep, wonderful voice of what you Feel inside, of your heart.* No longer tire yourself; don't exhaust yourself in thoughts or in deeds.

. . .

YOU ARE . . . NOW. You no longer RUN just anywhere in the desire to obtain something or get somewhere — whether it has to do with insisting on finishing a work or reaching a finish line or running the kilometers "someone" tells you is healthy. You no longer want to get "somewhere," no longer want to "endure," from your head, from your programmed *fixed ideas,* from your acquired convictions, because this destroys life. *You no longer insist on getting something "done," fixated in your head in a hard way: you let go and you arrive now at the essence of yourself, in love and mildness.* You now question everything and arrive at your true Heart: you learn to feel what life asks of YOU. Nothing is a "must". . . . Except "listening to this essential feeling of life," listening to your heart, to what your heart tells you is good for you.

Don't dwell on unimportant external factors or details. Live according to the essence . . . and Be who you ARE; remain always present with this BEING and don't "force" yourself into anything. Goodness and love count — not achieving, shining or responding to false ideals. Live and experience yourself in love, from the Core of your "I." Don't demand things from yourself . . . but LIVE out of the joy of your total, unified essence. Come into deeply felt contact with your heart, your body, your content of treasures. *You no longer force anything; you no longer want to obtain anything; therefore, you no longer get angry, in impatience or nervousness. You live out of goodness, in thankfulness for your being, looking at the Content, the Essence of things, people, life.*

Excerpt from the present book

About the symbolic meaning of "**glass that broke**" in the car accident: the synchronicity was patently obvious.

Suppressed POWERS ask for a conscious, constructive leadership: a resolute choice needs to be made. This will often imply a break with an old behavioral pattern, or literally making a break with an existing situation. A clear distinction has to be made between what is still possible and what isn't anymore, between good and bad. A definite SEPARATION of the wheat from the chaff needs to be accomplished. Something in you is "fighting" and asks for a solution. The inner struggle necessitates a settlement in favor of your good side.

Powers manifest themselves and need an UNEQUIVOQUAL, RESOLUTE CHOICE of the straight path, a break with a doubtful attitude: yes . . . no . . . . Employ these energies! Don't suppress anything; don't stand still, hesitating. Don't get angry but do what you have to do! Don't allow your powers to just roam around under your skin, in channels of indecision.

Your Living Self-Core refuses to continue in this way; the alarm bell is sounded.

. . .

Excerpt from *The Signal Book*[69]

He had felt for a long time that he had to quit his business, which was too much of a burden for him; but he kept wavering, yes / no, to quit / to continue. He didn't pay heed to the above-mentioned signals, nor to other ones, such as:

His sharp **shoulder pain**:

Fundamental Origin

Life weighs heavily on you: why do you burden yourself so? Why all these heavy worries? Does the anxiety press on your shoulders? You are bossy with yourself (perhaps also with others): you oblige yourself to do this or that, you "have to" do it; again and again you put up conditions for yourself in order for you to be able to accept yourself. You carry needless burdens: you block feelings and intuitive forces. You don't allow your nature to exist freely, flexibly, and relaxed!

You take burdens on your shoulders that are not at all necessary. Do you demand that you achieve or that you satisfy others? Do you want to manifest yourself as bigger and stronger than you inwardly feel? Do you ask too much of yourself? Misusing power regarding yourself? Don't you believe in your inner force, and do you therefore force yourself? Do you make yourself dependent on others? A feeling of powerlessness. Do you overload yourself with futilities, with details? Do relational problems weigh you down? Do you think, brood, so much?

---

[69] This work has not yet been published in English at the time of the publication of the present book.

Anxiety about the future: don't you trust life very much? You hurt yourself!

Fundamental Solution

Find the balance in yourself, and with a clear overview make your-self Master over your problems. Let go of all that is superfluous. Achieve no longer: accept yourself unconditionally. Your life is Joy if you create it yourself in a Self-aware way, if you no longer hold on to a Fate or an imaginary danger: you can direct your life, without misery. Discover this power of creation in yourself; intuitively follow your path; don't bottle up your feelings. You are good the way you are: feel safe and solid in the Basis of your deepest Self. Throw those needless burdens off your shoulders. Live spontaneously, free and happy, like a child.

Excerpt from *The Key to Self-Liberation*

His **painful neck**:

Fundamental Origin

Anxious stiffening: a feeling of inadequacy; you cannot or dare not completely "reach" things or confront yourself with them. You only look left or right, not daring to look in a wider scope. You feel "stuck," especially with regard to emotions. Your outer life-circumstances, the situations or things to which you stubbornly cling, are only a re-flection of your inner anxiety and unsureness.

Too stubborn, but especially too Afraid of "hearing" or "seeing": you flee.

You feel too small to take full responsibility; you feel unable to speak Straightforwardly, to be completely honest with yourself. Too afraid to bend; you flee from the truth regarding yourself.

You won't be able to position yourself in a flexible and open way because you don't really trust your inner Self. You tensely cling on to elements outside yourself, for support or security. You ignore your own authority.

Intense resistance, aggressive and stiff-necked behavior, a reac-tion to your inner powerlessness: this is how you demolish yourself, not allowing yourself to evolve flexibly. Obstinately holding fast to

your point of view without listening to facts that might mean enrich-
ment for you: Do you feel so threatened? You close yourself off
from your inner core of feeling, from your nature; you hold on to
needless tensions. You are too inflexible with yourself.

Fundamental Solution

Build your life on the guidance of your inner Authority and feel powerful in your Self. No longer flee from your inner wisdom and from
the message that others have for you: flexibly, and in a loving way,
open yourself to others. Listen to your feelings, to your nature: don't
force things, throw off needless burdens, let go of everything that
oppresses you.

In a self-assured way, determine your direction; direct yourself in
a flexible way at the path you intuitively feel is best, not allowing
yourself to be slowed down by suffocating, conservative thoughts
that hinder your evolution.

Excerpt from *The Key to Self-Liberation*
See also the other texts about the neck in the same book

In a long conversation with his friend, while resting on the couch, he
told about his fear of stopping his business: "And what then?" K. answered him that Life always asks to listen to "signals" such as symptoms and occurrences, and to act accordingly; that everything would
then work out fine; that one could not disregard this; and that when
you ignore these signals, then you will be confronted by ever stronger
signs from your life-core. N. quietly read the texts that applied to him:
about the chocolate that asked for softening, about the milk that indicated, among other things, "a new path to walk". . . .

"Yes, I have known it for a long time. I need to stop the business," N.
said.
K. answered him: "Life *allows* you to stop. You know that you create
your life yourself and that you always encounter the right thing on your
path — as long as you don't refuse to let go of the old, to listen to the
signals of life, of your own body. Don't worry, everything will be alright!"

While still reflecting and reading another time the texts about car accidents, heart arrhythmia, broken glass, etc., he saw a documentary on TV about the life of **beetles** and especially the **ladybird**. He vaguely remembered the texts in the book *If Animals Could Talk* and consulted the book again. He read about beetles and also about the deeper meaning of the ladybird. It touched him when he read that this little animal of fortune says: "Happiness lies in going onward! Don't look back anymore and you will be fine." But he had already made up his mind; the little red beetle only confirmed what he had read in the other texts that applied to him. It gave him inner peace. For the first time in months he did not sleep restlessly. He had taken his decision to quit his business and follow a new avenue. Heart arrhythmia disappeared gradually, his shoulders seemed to become lighter. Joy welled up inside him: because he had made the right choice on his path toward life.

The deeper meaning of the **ladybird** as described in the book *If Animals Could Talk*:

Like a discoverer exploring and liberating new grounds, making himself[70] master of them. Wiping the perspiration off his face every now and then, under his protective sun cap, and then going on unwearyingly, ever farther — on thin legs but strong, brave, and solid. Even if this requires a lot of effort, he keeps going onward for many days, not knowing when to stop. He doesn't even question this; he simply knows that he *has to* walk on. With this plucky, perseverant mentality he doesn't give up easily. He searches, examines, investigates. He shields himself from the sun although he can easily bear its rays.

. . .

His head is directed toward "the next thing." To put it in human language: his senses, his entire muscular and bone system already aim at going further, fully going onward toward a New Phase, again and again. He hates waiting too long. You might call him a little impatient; no, it's just that he is always ready to go further on the path he has chosen.

. . .

Time and again, he lets go of the previous thing and moves onward with powerful steps. His muscles tighten in order to clean up the old

---

[70] The author senses the ladybird as a masculine energy.

and go into the new. He sprints ahead and expels the old from his being. Sometimes with giant leaps, sometimes a little more quietly, but always with as much diligence and Aries Power. Dauntless. Everything that takes place in his head — his thoughts, his outlook on things, everything in his body — it all has to do with being hugely focused on dashing on, rolling on toward the next phase. He lives 'oriented toward the future'!
Everything at the service of this.

His message for Happiness to the Human Being?

This lovely little colorful beetle doesn't look back anymore and knows that his happiness lies in this: Unflinchingly going further onward, not letting himself be diverted by anything or anyone. Imperturbable, remaining on his Path. Opening up new possibilities, ever farther. Regularly enjoying delicious food, building up Force in him — with the eye always directed ahead.
. . .
"Push through to new domains," the lively little beetle adds, "go onward without hesitation and continue to further build up and develop your life."
. . .

Excerpt from the book If Animals Could Talk [71]

The man handed over his business and rested a couple of months before taking on a less demanding job for some years — with pleasure. He met the right people at the right places. Trust in the fact that life works that way, this is so important.

He is happy now. He only now completely realizes that nothing happens "just like that, by coincidence" — that everything has its meaning.

He had understood the messages of milk chocolate and milk, still happily and healthily enjoying their taste every so often — but the compulsive desire for large quantities of these food products had disappeared: because he had put into practice the admonitions he had been given through the language of these specific foodstuffs.

---

[71] This work has not yet been published in English at the time of the publication of the present book.

The new path of milk lay open to him. He didn't brood any longer and was entirely present in his earthly body. Gently, flexibly, and lovingly going onward as chocolate had asked him to do.

What about the Symbolic Language of Stars and Planets, Figures and Numbers, Trees and Animals?

It is not the stars and planets that determine our lives. At all times, we have our lives in our own hands.

Stars and planets all have their own "character," just as everything that lives has its own meaning, its own nature. In a birth chart (or horoscope) you can read with which convictions you have come into the world; *a horoscope does not reflect who and what you are in essence, but it reflects a whole world of convictions and, perhaps, behaviors that are a result of these convictions, which are deep inside yourself.* So, astrology is not meant to predict the future or to be dealt with in a superficial way, but it offers an interesting *Mirror Image* of the human being's convictions at the moment of his birth. It does need to be said that there exist several "levels" in human evolution, and therefore we have to deal with it in a very careful way. Still, this study of Stars and Planets in your birth chart is of importance if it's about finding the "thread of Ariadne." This information, after all, can help you more quickly get out of the Web in which you have held yourself imprisoned. For this reason, I have called up the deepest nature of 231 stars (from Sirius to Castor, etc.), and also the true meaning of why someone is born with the sun in the sign of Scorpio, Gemini, Capricorn, Leo, Sagittarius, etc.[72]

As long as Astrology is being used and studied in order to show the human being the way to "liberation," everything is okay. It's miraculous what characteristics every one of these stars carry inside them,

---

[72] Read about all this in *On Earth as in Heaven (The Psychological Language of the Fixed Stars),* in *Liberating Astrology (The deeper symbolism of the Sun in the signs of the Zodiac),* and in *The Black Moon and Priapus.* These books do not yet exist in English versions at the time of the publication of the present work.

and if one calculates a "star mirror" for a person,[73] then it's just as miraculous what philosophical psychological messages (signals) certain stars have to tell human beings: a colorful, instructive world!

Also, the symbolic meaning of "numbers" can learn us very much, in a compact, concentrated way. The wise human being opens himself up to it as well as to the symbolic values of stars and planets, of plants and animals and — not to be forgotten — of all the people around us. The greater the receptiveness of a human being who wants to know and search life more deeply, the easier will wealth and wisdom develop in him. But, remember: *it's neither the stars nor the numbers that "determine" your life. They just are mirrors or signs. ONLY YOU have your life, your future in hand!*

A lot of wisdom can be found in the primal symbolism of the different animal species. I wrote this down in *If Animals Could Talk.*[74] The giraffe, for instance, asks you not to forget the playful aspect in you. The mosquito pricks you so that you would be more awake in your life and live things more consciously. Etc. . . .

●

Illness: the Body speaks its own Language

The body speaks the language of our deepest Self. *The Key to healing and growth is true Insight into the psychological origin of illness or pain.* What we refer to as "illness" and pain are symptoms of inner disharmony, indications of the fact that something is not being realized — that something is not consciously known about one's own well-being. A psychological change will need to be brought about to cure the disorder. It's a good thing if the correct *insight* about this is acquired; practical application will follow. Neither conventional nor alternative medicine offer FUNDAMENTAL healing when they overlook the *psy-*

---

[73] The "Star-mirror" — which stars make an aspect with certain planets in your birth chart?

[74] This work has not yet been published in English at the time of the publication of the present book.

chological correction which needs to be done in order for the body to continue healing itself in an autonomic way. Take away the psycho-emotional origin and the symptom disappears.

Of course, classical or natural medicine can be taken in this transitional phase of humankind, in case of illness or moments of crisis; this won't have a negative effect on the human being on the condition *that one work simultaneously on the true, fundamental, psycho-emotional origins of the problem.* (Please read more about this in the chapter: "Arrive at healing with or without remedies from the outside.")

Infection and Contagion

Infections are (at the physical level) caused by micro-organisms: by viruses, fungi, bacteria. These organisms are constantly teeming in, on, and around our body, even when we are healthy. *We are by nature immune* to "contagion," to "developing illness" from one of these elements — immune to whatever negative influence by whatever organism. Earth swarms with thousands of types of bacteria, which by themselves are all harmless.

Certain people can be in close contact with contagious diseases for no matter how long or how intense, and still they will not be infected, while others will get sick right away. It does not matter if we are dealing here with a common cold, tuberculosis, or AIDS. *What is the real origin of contagion, of infections?* How do we stay healthy?

Certain feelings — i.e. anxiety, aggression, grudge, etc. — thoughts, and convictions activate that specific virus inside you, touch that specific body part of yours that best corresponds with this specific *dislocation of your psyche, your convictions,* . . . .

The book *The Key to Self-Liberation* explains what kind of dislocation corresponds to any specific illness. There's no question whatsoever of feeling guilty about this; the point is to bring about changes in your psycho-emotional system.

When people with similar soul-states (for instance feelings of inferiority) meet each other, then they will be more susceptible to "infecting" each other.

Your unconscious and conscious longings, your thinking patterns and your emotions, your convictions and expectations of life — these determine your body cells, your organs, your glands, your hormonal changes; determine your susceptibility to contagion.

True contagiousness is to be found in your own psychological pattern, which can then be even enhanced by the transfer of negative convictions from generation to generation, from father to son, from doctor to patient.

Becoming aware of the endless *possibilities* for growth and healing in the human being would be an important Step forward which Medical Science would do well to take.

Arrive at Healing:
with or without Remedies from the Outside?

Without remedies from the outside?

Many have already shown that it is possible to arrive at healing without remedies from the outside: by solving the true origins of the illness, the psycho-emotional fundamental reason why the illness was able to come to be.

Read the sections in *The Key to Self-Liberation* that are relevant to the symptoms or illnesses you are plagued with — read slowly and attentively, and come to an intense realization of the "why," to INSIGHT into the deepest origin that has enabled the disease to develop in you. Then, read the incentive to the fundamental solution and put it into practice in your daily life.

One person needs more time for this than another; in one person there's stronger resistance, or a more chronic process going on than in another person. Everyone will bring about healing at their own tempo, in their very own way. **But most people are not ready for effecting healing without conventional medicine**.

Therefore, don't take any risk in case of serious diseases; don't stubbornly refuse conventional medical treatment when you have a need for medicine, therapies, surgery, etc. We may be thankful that these remedies exist in our time. This is no coincidence either.

With remedies from the outside

When, in this phase of transition, in a certain stage of psychological development, or during a moment of crisis, one calls upon medicine or other remedies from the outside (such as surgery, etc.), then Life inside you finds this to be okay. Do not at all feel guilty about this! You are allowed to make it easier for yourself; you don't have to suffer pain, and it's perfectly alright if at certain moments you use remedies from the outside, ON THESE CONDITIONS:

1) *That in the meantime you work on the TRUE, fundamental causes, psycho-emotionally, which brought on your illness.* If you don't do this, then merely making use of medicine or methods — *whether conventional or alternative methods of treatment* — means that you suppress Signals that your Living Self is sending you in order to make something very clear to you: changes need to be made Inside you, in your existence.

   If you ignore these symptoms and just heal them with natural medicine or allopathic methods, without in the meantime working on the deeper origins, then you are not *truly* healed. Sooner or later, your Life-Core will send a new illness to you — so that you now begin to work on the *true* cause of your illness symptom. The purpose of your Living Self is ultimately to bring you ever more strongly on the path of true life, in truth, toward greater happiness. Therefore, listen to it, no matter if you use remedies or not.

2) That one doesn't become *dependent* on the remedy in such a way that — in a prolonged process through which a sort of *"laziness"* develops — that, finally, you might lose all faith in your own self-healing powers. At that moment you might have to check yourself, depend more upon yourself, and *strengthen the faith* in your inner self-healing abilities. After all, healing methods from the outside remain only expedients that have nothing to do with the CORE of the problem. They can assist you for a while, but in the end YOU heal yourself "in the core." Medicine can only be called a temporary aid and won't do it instead. Only you can realize **fundamental** healing, as described earlier in this book.

3) *That, in the meantime, you understand that you give yourself this remedy with love, but that it is really you who will heal you.* After

all, you can take whatever remedy, but the healing only will be true and definitive if you "inwardly" set to work on yourself and adjust your course. Then, it is not the remedy that will have cured you — it was and is only a help. You have then healed yourself and your Living Self-Core doesn't need to send you another signal anymore. As *Master* over your life, you have given yourself an aid, (the remedy), without feeling "addicted." You have given it to yourself lovingly, and you stop giving it when it is good to stop.

No matter whether it's about allopathy, acupuncture, flower therapy, diet therapy, homeopathy, etc., it is not at all wrong or bad to make use of them. But essentially these could be considered as artificial interventions from the outside, by which one actually doubts the self-healing nature of a human being. This is, however, very understandable in the light of the gradual process, of evolution and becoming aware, which the human being and humankind are going through.

The time has to be ripe. The human being grows by *communicating lovingly with himself.* When he is afraid, not really sure, convinced to be unable to manage without remedies from the outside, or when he is not yet ready for this in his evolution process — as is still the case with many people today — then, in loving communication with himself, in and through his deepest self-core, he will feel and know that in his deepest life essence it is accepted and understood that he temporarily uses natural or conventional remedies from the outside. Yes, of course this is allowed . . . and finally, it is intended that in his life process the human being eventually feels that he no longer needs any remedies or help at all from the outside. It is not until the apple is ripe that it falls from the tree.

Do not force anything to happen before its time. Do not condemn yourself if you cannot do without remedies from the outside yet; do not force yourself to succeed without help. Even the wisest, strongest people on earth can deem it advisable to make use of, for instance, medicine or a surgical intervention at a certain time in their lives. This is no sign of weakness.

Numerous people recover, without medicine, from all kinds of illnesses, from the most innocuous to the most serious; others feel they have to make use of remedies. One's own conviction, one's own faith, and the phase of evolution or transformation in which one is, play the leading role here, and it's important that one listen to this. Of course I, as the author, do not bear any responsibility for your choice.

Therefore: this book does not say: "Throw away all medicine and other remedies." It shows you the underlying origins of illnesses, and that an illness is only truly "healed" when those origins are resolved, no matter if the healing has been effected with or without help from the outside.

In principle, it can be done without remedies, as many have already shown, but here, *you should do as you feel and not be hard on yourself.* Also, don't take any risk. If, during a difficult period, you feel you need a calming pill or herbal tincture, then take it. Be gentle to yourself . . . ON THE CONDITION that in the meantime you work on the causes of your depression, nervous breakdown, etc.[75] Medication, operations, radiotherapy, chemotherapy, etc.: make use of them when you have the feeling that it's good to do so. Talk about this with competent doctors who also know the connection between body and psyche.

The person who already *truly* knows and feels: "I BELIEVE, I can and will heal myself without remedies from the outside," will indeed be able to bring this into realization — if this is his autonomous decision, and not "because he read it in *The Key to Self-Liberation* and just will give it a try." For such things are felt and decided deep within one's "I." Also, as pointed out before, the person needs to *really* understand and thoroughly resolve the psycho-emotional problem that underlies his ailments. *Here, every human being needs to accept his own responsibility and know,* feel deep inside, whether he is ready for this, without building upon other people's theories while doing so. Don't take any risk.

All the cells of your body are constantly being influenced by your emotions, your thoughts, your convictions. If you have complete confidence in your body, then every cell, every element of your body, will feel good and will execute its task optimally.

Minor illnesses ask for a minor, but not unimportant, change in your life. Don't suppress them right away with remedies. First of all, try to find out why you have a headache, throat ache, stomach ache, or inflammation. After all, if you immediately suppress these symptoms

---

[75] Consult the relevant chapters in *The Key to Self-Liberation*.

with medicines or think you have no other choice than, for instance, to build up your immunity via herbal extracts or homeopathy, then you don't really believe in your Ability, in your built-in, innate, very powerful Immune System. (Read more in *The Key to Self-Liberation* under the category "AIDS.") Then, you make yourself totally dependent on remedies from the outside, while everything is really inside you.

Immunity is inside you: an illness, no matter which one, disappears — the body recovers naturally — if you *truly* and fundamentally take away the PSYCHOLOGICAL ORIGIN. Your body indicates what needs to be changed in your life in order to live in greater Happiness and harmony. From this perspective, illness is a blessing; but being sick is not *necessary* for evolution. No one has to suffer: you, as a human being, have everything in hand.[76] Arrive at deeper insight, at deep Self-Love. Know that, when it's necessary to take them, painkillers don't just exist by chance. As long as you don't misuse them and thankfully offer yourself this soothing of pain.

Insight and Ignorance
Becoming Aware

Our deepest, or true, Living Self-Core, this immortal Self, is the wellspring of our existence. It directs our life. We may trust in it completely, without anxieties. It leads us to an earthly existence if we carry that longing inside us. We are born *there,* in that milieu, with these life circumstances which best give us a reflection of our *inner convictions* or our *expectations for our life.* We are not born here or there out of a "conscious" choice: nobody, after all, would then be born in miserable circumstances. *A sad environment at birth or a handicap does not indicate a "punishment from God," nor does it indicate a "Karma" that one would have deserved as a consequence of so-called bad deeds in a previous life. It simply indicates the web in which we are psychologically imprisoned. It simply indicates the convictions deep inside ourselves.* If it's our conviction that we are poor victims or sinners, who are only allowed to suffer and do penance — unable to take their lives into their own hands in a self-aware manner, but think that life should be put into the hands of one or another god or of a Destiny —

---

[76] See the text "Immune Deficiency Diseases" in *The Key to Self-Liberation — Encyclopedia of Psychosomatics.* Don't be overconfident but steadily evolve onward.

then we unconsciously choose a sad, powerless, slave existence. Misery in the world is the consequence of a shortage of Insight and an abundance of "Unawareness" and ignorance. That's why humankind has every reason to lead itself toward "Consciousness."

The kind of life we are living, the illnesses we "get," are a consequence of our inner convictions and psychological patterns. *In proportion to the human being's increasing Awareness of his responsibility, of his possibilities to create his own life, a new world can be born.*

Beyond Einstein:
Consciousness Energy Governs Matter

Life is no coincidence. Nothing happens "just like that." Yet nothing is "fixed," nothing is predestined. Science already knows *that energy and matter are interchangeable,* but often one isn't yet aware of one step further that needs to be taken; it is forgotten that all energy represents "a kind of life-consciousness." The conversion of energy into matter actually happens by the inner driving force of this "life-consciousness" that lies behind it. Our body exists thanks to the inner "Life-Consciousness."

So, if we exit the unaware phase and if we **CONSCIOUSLY direct our life-energies in goodness** — while understanding the signals that life shows us or lets us experience, and consequently bringing about the necessary changes — then the world transforms totally. We only need to be aware of it, to do it! Consciousness energies influence matter. Therefore, the human being and humanity do well to consciously and lovingly make use of them in order to create a happy world, a healthy body.

●

There is no hell, not here, nor after death, unless we create one ourselves, by anxiety, by our frustrations and by our negative imaginings and expectations. Illness and misery — in the world, and individually — are caused by the fact that we are cut off from our Living Self, from our imperishable nucleus, our wellspring.

Deep within us rage negative opinions about ourselves: Do you think yourself inferior or bad? Then your Living Self will send out signals via the body (for example, migraines[77]), then it will also attract situations in life which mirror your convictions (for instance a father or a partner who belittles you).

Never condemn others. You have attracted to yourself, albeit unconsciously, certain people and circumstances that present a looking glass for your inner convictions. Change your opinion, your philosophy of life, and the convictions about yourself. As a consequence, the circumstances around you will change. What illness do you have? What does your body tell you about yourself? Did you, albeit unconsciously, call up a "fall," and are you stuck with a bone fracture? Then look hard inside yourself: you want to break out of something, you are rebelling. Etc. . . .[78] Discover the true cause.

The body is constantly being formed by the Living Self: if we trust in our Source, then we allow energies to flow freely, also the healing powers. Immunity means, among other things: Trust in our Source, which constantly holds growth and health. It means going along with the flow of your life, trusting in the Inner Power, in self-authority, taking joy in your existence, feeling love for yourself. Knowing that this divine nucleus, this primal urge for life propels us onward, again and again, in spontaneous creativity and unlimited mobility, leading us to an ever-greater fulfillment, consciousness, raising the value of our life.

We human beings are all on our way.

A surrender to our Living Self, self-creating life, a balance between common sense, the rational mind on the one hand and the intuition and feelings on the other hand. Such a strong faith in immunity, in the possibility of having our health in our own hands, that no illness can penetrate. Fears disappear when we trust in our Self, when we realize that we can create our own existence; we will not Want or Force happenings to take place, but we can call up these happenings in our life which are the best for us and for our fellow human beings. Take the rudder of life solidly in your hands!

---

[77] See the chapter about migraine in *The Key to Self-Liberation*.
[78] See the chapters about bone fractures in *The Key to Self-Liberation*.

Don't Confuse "Positive Thinking" with "Desiring in Thought" or "Wanting to Grab"

It is self-evident that it is better to think positively than negatively. Yet, neither positive thinking nor positive visualizing nor looking in the mirror every day and saying, "I become better and better every day" have any positive effect if deep inside yourself there exists a contrary **conviction**, such as, "I know I cannot do that; I was not born to be happy; I do not deserve it; I am undoubtedly a nothing, etc." You may stand in front of the mirror as much as you want and say, "I am beautiful, I am strong," but if you do not solve the deeper cause of your sadness and your illness, and you remain convinced of "I am weak and ugly," then positive thinking has no purpose.

True creation happens, first and foremost, *via the elimination of negative, unconscious convictions and expectations regarding yourself and life. This will enable you to create your life in a self-aware way, on a positive basis.*

When you think positively — "I *must* and will have that job. I *have* to be taken on by this company." — then you may think as much as you want, but if this job is not good for you at this moment, then you won't get it. In this case, don't force things. *Don't desire (grab) with thoughts. On the contrary, it is better to say: "I am convinced I will find the most ideal job with regard to nature, time, content, and place,"* and the rest you leave open. No fatalism, but a positive creating, and being open at the same time to what is best for you at the moment. Yes, just open yourself up to everything that is being offered: you look in newspapers, you talk to people who don't simply appear on your path "by coincidence." For the rest, have faith in your Living Self, in your inner computer, which knows very well what's good for you, and this is not always what you (Here is meant: the thinking, desiring "Little I") WANT.

Are you sick, then you'd better ask yourself: "What is the cause of my illness?" "Why does my Living Self send signals?" There is no point in screaming, "I Will and Shall get better," when in the meantime you don't understand the meaning and the language of your illness. Read again, in *The Key to Self-Liberation,* the texts that apply to you. Talk about it with someone who knows you very well, or with a competent doctor or health professional who can comprehend your psychosomatic issues. Listen to your body; ask your Living Self for psychological enlightenment, and you will attract circumstances which are a result of your call to understand your illness. Solve the psychological problem which lies behind it, and so recuperative forces coming from your Living Self are activated.

Also, concerning money and material possessions: it's of no use to direct your thoughts particularly toward this. Let go! Trust, and know that life gives you at every moment what's good for you.[79]

Be careful not to use Thought Forces as a means of Power

Whether it's about positive or negative thoughts, carefully avoid using them as a means of power, no matter if they are directed toward yourself or others. *For in these cases, one often neglects to very consciously carry out changes in the fundamental, psycho-emotional origins of illnesses,* or to reflect on the why of this or that unpleasant occurrence which one has attracted in one's life.

Healing sometimes takes some time, even though it can go fast; it needs to run PARALLEL to the steps forward one takes, the necessary psycho-emotional changes one carries through in oneself. One will do well not to force things by thought forces or, for instance, by drastic hypnosis sessions — neither with regard to illnesses nor with regard to occurrences, because these are all signals. Learn to distinguish the chaff from the wheat with respect to health professionals. And aspire to purity, to integrity, in yourself.

Create Your Own Life

Wish, long, produce thoughts, express your wishes, call it up, very consciously — and then wait trustingly. Meanwhile, your environment gives you signs when you go wrong, for you also have attracted this environment, be it unconsciously. Or, your body will tell you via sig-

---

[79] The true origin of "financial problems" can be solved at the core just by positive thinking (read about this in *The Signal Book*) and doesn't ask for a positive "calling up" of money.

nals or via an illness where you are wrong, for your Living Self uses your body as "language." Do not resist what your body or circumstances tell you, and go along smoothly to where you feel your Self is leading you. Let go where you feel you have to let go: a sign that something new in your life will be born. Your Living Self, "you" in fact are it, listen to it; an ever greater Unity will result.

The melting together of the Human Being and the divine in him will give rise to a more Self-Aware being, who is taking his life and his body in his own hands. It will lead him to still unknown perspectives, to a new body, and if he wishes to earthly immortality[80] and exploration of other worlds.

Children

In the present stage of evolution of humankind, children are born by mothers.

The human being is born with certain expectations, certain anxieties, certain hopeful outlooks on life. Anyhow, the human being will be born there, where he will find a reflection of his negative as well as positive expectations and convictions regarding himself and life in general. He manifests himself in his body in a unique way.

Children are no-one's possessions, not the parents' nor the upbringers'. They belong to themselves. Therefore, give them to the life in themselves.

Children are not born anywhere "just by chance." Their Living Self-Core brings or drives them in this direction, to those parents, in that milieu — where a mirror is held up to them. Here, with this genetic, basic material (which in evolution is susceptible to transformation), in this environment and with these people as upbringers. This is a point of departure on earth which the being — be it unconsciously — has attracted on the basis of its convictions, its expectations regarding life, its nature. Life circumstances reflect the inner state the child is born with.

---

[80] Read more about this in *New Days*. This work has not yet been published in English at the time of the publication of the present book.

The baby, who is born with certain psychological patterns has "come" to these specific upbringers in order, via confrontation, to give a solution to these problems.

Babies and children are very easily influenced by, and very sensitive to, mental signals which are being sent out, be it unconsciously, by people with whom they have close ties. Let us take throat infection as an example;[81] we will find the same psychological meaning, and perhaps will find it even stronger with the mother and/or father. Here, angry, powerless, fearful emotions should be resolved by mother / father and child.

There is no question of guilt here, for the child was born — with certain psychological disharmonies — to precisely these parents, so that, via confrontations, it can solve these psycho-emotional issues. The parent, in her or his turn, can evolve by examining him/herself in the face of the reflection that the little one is for him/her. Mother resolves, for instance, her powerless anger and thereby helps the baby as well as herself by bringing about changes in her inner situation via clear insight and by putting this insight into practice in her daily life. This can have a positive influence on the recovery of both.

When parents or upbringers become aware of the psycho-emotional undercurrents of an ailment in the baby, then this already enables them to approach the baby in the right manner — on the basis of these insights. This allows the healing process to have its first beginning. One can make things clear to young children much earlier than one thinks. Communication and ability to sense.

One needs to emphasize *that the deepest* **origin** *of the illness always needs to be looked for in the psycho-emotional state of the child itself.* Although the stronger the tie between parent and child, the stronger the factor of influence from parent to child on the psychological level.

The more independent and autonomous the child becomes while growing up, the more this factor will disappear. Then it will no longer be true that "parent(s) and child are like mirrors to one another" on whatever level, including the image of illnesses or ailments. Everyone would do well to faithfully follow his or her own nature; no-one needs to follow in someone else's footsteps. Everyone has his or her own path of evolution to travel. It's a good thing that parents or upbringers

---

[81] Please read more about throat conditions in *The Key to Self-Liberation*.

give guidance and information. Of course, unhealthy interference or tyrannical coercion toward children needs to be avoided. After all, the child also needs its "experiences"; it's a good thing if the child finds its personal, highly unique path. Conversely, Life also requires respect and understanding from the children for parents or upbringers who mean well.

It is of utmost importance to the young people that upbringers or parents are a noble *example* to them — loving, full of integrity, growing by becoming aware.

Let us hereby ask whether the "system" humankind has created — the "bearing of children" (mostly going together with painful labor), bringing "powerless" beings into the world, beings who, if not fed by the parents, would die — whether this "system" is the most ideal. *Would it be better to create a world* where there is no question of dependency, powerlessness, pain — ever and again starting "anew" on a relatively "unconscious" level?

House Pets

Pets receive the positive as well as the negative psycho-emotional, electromagnetic radiations from their "master." They are very sensitive to the alternating changes in the affective world of their masters. No matter if it concerns a dog, a horse, a bird, or a cat, they will be a reflection of that which is in disharmony in you.

Does your dog suffer from knee joint pain? Look in *The Key to Self-Liberation*, then, under the section about the knee, and you will find the psychological origins to be present in yourself, as the master. A message from the dog to its master. Listen to these natural messages and make the necessary changes in your life. In this way you help each other. What has been said before about "children" can also be applied here.

It is often said that dog and master "resemble" each other; and that is so. It is not "just by chance" that a pet with a specific character ends up with you. Yet, as with children, the ORIGIN of the illness always lies in the being (the animal), itself. The master, or upbringer, never has any "guilt" regarding his pet's illness. He can, however, positively influence the healing process by bringing about changes in himself, as the upbringer. After all, it is not for nothing that he "attracts" the situation of his house pet having an ailment, as a "reflection" of something in him.

Becoming Aware and Responsibility

Our body, matter, exist only because of and thanks to the inner Power source, which can be considered to be the motor of our life. The individualized spirit which reveals itself in matter.

It is necessary that we grow toward more *self-awareness,* to a stronger Faith in our possibilities, to unconditional Love for ourselves; that, like proud commanders of the ship of life, we know an immortal nucleus lies deep inside us, which immediately sends us signals when we deviate from the right course, so that we can redirect our lives, in a Conscious way.

We are not subject to unconscious urges anymore, to unconscious passions, to instincts, we do not let ourselves "be lived" . . . whenever we do not wish so, whenever, with the Conscious "I," we direct our creative forces and deep natural feelings in the light of a future which we ourselves can build. We are not victims unless we doom ourselves to it.

The world will stay full of misery if we do not believe in our own creative power, if we keep on waiting for a rescue from the outside, if we keep on pointing the judgmental finger at others. The building of a beautiful planet, without illness, without war, starts with Belief, Becoming Aware, and Love.

To make others aware begins with becoming aware yourself.

Be the *master* of your life, your body. Solve the psycho-emotional issues that underlie possible illnesses or other symptoms; as a result, self-healing powers will be stimulated. Build up the intense Love for yourself. Believe in yourself and be open to the *true* origins of your illness — while being patient with yourself. Always keep going onward, full of trust; in the meantime bring about the necessary changes in yourself step by step. Life will assist you!

Do not fanatically exclude any doctor or health professional. Communication is salutary.

Building an "Earthly Paradise"

Life has placed "spiritual consciousness energies" into "Matter," and by so doing has given birth to the planet Earth, to the Human Being. Thus, Life has established the basis for further growth — for possibilities which ultimately will result in a paradisaical situation.

It is via the Earth and the Human Being that Life wishes to continuously construct and develop itself in the richest possible way. We shouldn't be looking for paradise outside the earthly spheres, in other dimensions — even if these other dimensions interpenetrate with our earthly spheres. We as human beings will do well — beginning with "Life in Matter" as the secure basis upon which we can build — to create a paradisaical sphere. An ideal, marvelous fusion within our "I" of "spiritual consciousness" and "physical experience" — here on Earth!

Let us **make an eternal Alliance with Life**, everyone individually, in order to make something magnificent of it.

Life counts on us, and we as human beings have the responsibility of bringing Life itself to further growth and fulfillment "according to living perspectives," on Earth.

Happiness lies in our hands: a possibility of "creating" given us by Life, crystallized in our Living Self, brimming with the power of faith and the energy of love. These enormous potentialities lie in the human being who indeed attunes to "True Life" in thankfulness for his "Being," as "I." It's up to this Human Being to DO it, to work on the Building of a Paradise: in himself, on Earth. Don't wait for someone else, for "something" else. *You, consciously living Human Being, believe in yourself, and do it! For Life, for the Earth, for Yourself, for all People who are full of love.*

From the HERE-AND-NOW
You Can Create Your Life —
Not from Yesterday or Tomorrow or Elsewhere

Everything is energetically interconnected. The world is not energetically divided into pigeon-holes. Certain energies attract each other, others reject each other. When you live with positive expectations regarding your life — in the here-and-now! — then you attract all that is beautiful: that which is good for you.

Directing your energies, leading your life: this is only possible from the HERE-AND-NOW. Not from yesterday, not from the thought of tomorrow, not from a place where you are not present NOW.

Therefore, it is very important to always stay "with yourself" in the here-and-now. Don't fly away in thoughts and dreams, to memories from the past, to possibilities in the future, to distant countries or imaginary places.

And *if* at a certain moment the past or the future do become a topic of conversation or thought, then meanwhile, stay IN YOUR BODY, with both feet on the ground. Stay consciously present in the here-and-now.

Your dreams and thoughts are not master over you; it's just the other way around! Fantasy, imagination, thoughts, . . . are all alright, but only under the sovereignty of your Awareness: your awareness of being here and now, as master of your life, strongly grounding your spirit in your earthly body.

In this way you can regenerate and heal faster.

Thankfulness:
the Key toward Life in Happiness

And . . . have you got off the right track for a moment? Do you not see a way out anymore? Then tune yourself to THANKFULNESS again. Thankfulness for YOUR BEING, because you have been given the privilege to BE, to exist, as a Human Being on Earth. Acknowledge your unique being, your value.

In this vibration of gratitude, Life itself will help you — Life deep inside you, because you have connected yourself again with this wavelength which gives life and brings happiness.

Therefore: *"Thank you, Life, that I exist, that I have been given the opportunity to 'be,' as 'I' on Earth!"* In this way the opening is freed for the flow of joy in your being, and also for the delightful happenings which you can, and will, encounter on your path, "not just by chance," very soon.

●

FUNDAMENTAL ORIGINS AND SOLUTIONS FOR ILLNESSES,
on the Psychological-Emotional Level

PSYCHOLOGICAL SYMBOLISM
OF PARTS OF THE BODY ·

Insights about Emotions, Psychological Phenomena,
the Authentic Body Shape, Genetic Patterns, etc.

●

Texts that were added or thoroughly revised
for the Second Edition of the Book
"The Key to Self-Liberation® — Encyclopedia of Psychosomatics"

CORONAVIRUS

First, it is very important to underline that in the text hereafter there's no question whatsoever of "guilt or fault." One does *not* get SARS or CoViD-19 because of "guilt, punishment, or penance."

From out of a heartfelt concern for all the suffering resulting from CoViD-19 — and hand in hand with medical science — the present text aims to stimulate the human being to **become aware** of certain (often unconscious) psychological patterns, emotional states, habits, convictions, beliefs, instinctive tendencies, a tarnished self-image, etc., that are not beneficial. Thanks to awareness-raising one can, if one wishes, try to change these patterns in oneself.

The group of coronaviruses has been known for many decades (together with rhinoviruses, adenoviruses, enterovirus-es, etc.) as viruses that cause harmless colds. In some colds such a (harmless) coronavirus can be the responsible a-gent. People who have symptoms of a common cold, brought about by any germ, can read the relevant texts in the book *The Key to Self-Liberation – Encyclopedia of Psychosomatics:* common cold, running nose, stuffy nose, sneezing, sore throat, tearing eyes, sinusitis, etc.

In 2002-2003 the so-called **SARS** epidemic broke out in Asia. The responsible agent was a *new* coronavirus, called SARS-CoV-**1**, which, in addition to flu-like symptoms, could cause severe pneumonia and even death. SARS stands for "Severe Acute Respiratory Syndrome." In 2012, the so-called MERS disease, triggered by another *new* coronavirus, broke out in the Middle East.

At the end of 2019 the so-called **CoViD-19** epidemic broke loose in China (CoViD-19 = **Co**rona **Vi**rus **D**isease 20**19**). In the following months CoViD-19 spread all over the world (= pandemic). The coronavirus responsible for CoViD-19, called SARS-CoV-**2**, is genetically very similar to SARS-CoV-**1** which was responsible for SARS.

By the end of March 2020, a number of scientists said that the new coronavirus is almost the same virus as the one that had caused SARS, but that small mutations would have made it less deadly but more contagious. (One can be contagious to others without showing symptoms.) In medical practice, doctors would not be able to distinguish between the syndromes of SARS and CoViD-19. So CoViD-19 and SARS would actually be the same disease, according to these scientists.

Have you become infected with the coronavirus of CoViD-19? Then all the necessary information about the psychological-emotional breeding ground for the virus is in this book and in *The Key to Self-Liberation*. This information can make you aware of certain patterns in yourself. Hand in hand with expert medical help you can try and change these patterns in yourself, in order to solve the psychological-emotional origin in yourself. This is called fundamental healing.

With the coronavirus, life has given you a *signal*. By awareness-raising through the texts in this book and in *The Key to Self-Liberation* — and by putting this into practice in your daily life — you listen to what this signal has to tell you. In this way, there needn't be a new signal in the future that means the same thing.

In this respect, what are the relevant texts? It depends on the symptoms that this coronavirus has caused in you.

Do you experience only mild symptoms, like those of a common cold? Then read the related texts (as indicated above for the "harmless" coronaviruses).

Is it as if you have the flu? Then read in this book, and/or in *The Key to Self-Liberation,* the texts about flu, fever, muscular pain, cough. . . .

Do you suffer from loss of smell or taste? Diarrhea? Headaches? Anxiety? These texts can also be found in *The Key to Self-Liberation*.

Other important texts are about infections in general, inflammation in general, penetration of a virus, air and airways.

Also page 5 to 118 of this book, especially chapters like "Infection and Contagion," "Illness: the Body speaks its own Language," "Illness as a Signal," etc.

Have you become seriously ill? Or, have you even been admitted to an intensive care unit? Then be sure to read and deeply understand the texts about SARS, pneumonia, shortness of breath (and, possibly, also the texts about thrombosis, embolism, coagulation disorders, kidney failure, etc.).

Are you healthy, but are you afraid of being infected?

Of course it is important that you observe the precautions and measures that the medical experts and the authorities announce.

In addition, an attentive reading of the chapters in this book — and in *The Key to Self-Liberation* — about flu, SARS, pneumonia, anxiety, can be worthwhile. Take a look deep inside and examine thoroughly to what extent these texts apply to you. Then endeavor to do something about it.

This is an additional way to try and remove the breeding ground for the virus as much as possible. You can only benefit from this.

In *The Key to Self-Liberation,* it is also interesting to read the following texts: Immune Deficiency, Respiratory Tract, and Lungs, in general.

What is the meaning of CoViD-19 for the world, for humanity?

The 1918-1919 flu pandemic (influenza) killed many millions. Nowadays, the threat of bird flu (fowl plague) and other epidemics also remains very real. Medical researchers work to develop, and discover, all kinds of vaccines and treatments, which of course is an excellent thing.

At the same time, there is the psychological-emotional undercurrent that corresponds to the fact that influenza and corona viruses can enter a human body and use human cells to multiply, causing these cells to be destroyed.

Dealing with this psychological-emotional undercurrent, this "fundamental origin" of flu, and also of SARS and CoViD-19, as described in the present work, can only be realized by each human being individually.

Self-examination, becoming aware, and endeavoring to put this into practice — every human being is completely free to choose this path or not.

Every human being is free to believe or not to believe that there is a psychological-emotional origin for illness, and that one can try to solve this in oneself.

In 2020, we see on a global scale that only a very small minority of people are prepared to look **INSIDE** themselves in order to go in search of the fundamental psychological origin of this or that disease.

Life, or the Source of Life, has for centuries sent out the signal of flu, in order that every human being would understand and change certain essential things in himself: all details can be found in the texts mentioned above.

2020 brings the message of CoViD-19 that has many similar symptoms as the flu, but a higher percentage of serious or fatal cases. It's as if Life has now called up "flu with a giant exclamation mark."

A harbinger was SARS in 2003. The 2020 CoViD-19 pandemic shakes the foundations of the whole of humanity. Will there be people who will now take a serious look inside themselves, in search of the deeper meaning of flu and SARS???

Could it be that not a single person in the world has completely understood the above-mentioned psychological, emotional, metaphysical origin of flu, SARS, and CoViD-19 in himself? That no-one on earth has already put into practice the essential solution?

Hence the importance of becoming aware — ever more strongly and deeply — of the "why." Every human being can only realize this in himself. Everyone is free to believe this or not, to try and deal with this within themselves or not.

In the meantime one should be very grateful for the help that medical science can provide. Undoubtedly new vaccines, new antiviral drugs, new health measures will be elaborated in order to overcome CoViD-19, and that's a very good thing.

But after that??? Do we just wait until the next new virus pops up? Or do we choose the path of "looking inward, inside ourselves"? By using the texts about SARS and flu given to us by Christiane Beerlandt? Trying to understand the deeper "why"? And putting this into practice in our own lives? Every human being has the choice.

Some Reflections

Signals keep bubbling up out of the Well-spring of Life in order that the human being would put himself more and more on the wavelength of "Life," the energy of "*truly* living." Away from "death" and everything that vibrates on the wavelength of "death."

At the same time, new impulses, initiatives, discoveries, strategies, insights, awakenings, . . . sprout from the human being himself. They contribute to the fact that humankind and the planet Earth can continue to exist, while evolving toward ever more fulfilment and harmony, toward ever new possibilities.

This can only work with Love as a basis.

Flu (influenza) means "inflow" or "influence"; corona means "crown." People who choose to do so can now put the lessons of coronavirus into practice; in this way they take steps forward, on the road to a coronation: the human being elevates himself to an ever more noble, conscious, loving level.

The corona pandemic has brought about major changes in society. In fact, the human being is pushing himself toward the solution as described in Christiane Beerlandt's texts about flu and SARS. Even on an unconscious level, many are taking steps in this direction.

Now let the whirligig, the jumble, the hustle, the crisscross, the bedlam calm down.

The human being will do well to quiet his HEAD, his feverish thoughts, his bustling.

Let the human being nestle peacefully and delightfully in his own body, like a purring cat near a cozy stove. Smelling nature again, tasting its fruits, taking the time to appreciate.

Not "desiring" all the time to go to all kinds of places in order to "fill" oneself with stimuli, people, and things, from the outside.

Digitization, internet, computer games, social media, TV series, films, gambling, devices such as smartphones, tablets, etc., virtual worlds. . . . There are many advantages to the digital age that can help humanity. But if one loses oneself completely in all this (for instance, while one is obliged to stay at home for several weeks or months), then does one listen enough to the signal of flu and CoViD-19?

When one forces 70-80-90-. . . year-olds to go digital — with all the stressful situations and loss of warm personal contacts this can entail for these people — then does one do that which flu and CoViD-19 ask from humankind?

Wouldn't it be necessary to respect "limits of humanity" amidst the digital craze?

Besides human viruses there are also computer viruses. The psychological-emotional state of a person whose computer is infected by a virus is described by Christiane Beerlandt in *The Signal Book.*[1]

People who live "alone" are more intensely confronted with this "living alone."

This is an opportunity to strongly attune oneself to the only true source of joy and love, which resides deeply **IN** oneself.

---

[1] This work hasn't yet been translated into English at the time of the publication of the present book.

Autonomy. Arriving at a sense of gratitude for the miracle of one's own "being," independent of anyone or anything else.

People who live "together" are more intensely confronted with this "living together."

This is an opportunity to learn to fall back strongly on one's own basis — the rock-solid foursquare structure that is automatically a marked-off personal terrain of which no-one else can violate the boundaries unasked.

Learning to understand each other's nature and limits. Communication in mutual respect.

Do you feel trapped in too small a space? Experience the grandiose space of your inner world, the vastness of your personal content.

If needed, see the solution to claustrophobia in *The Key to Self-Liberation*.

Whether living alone or in a group, everyone attracts the experiences he or she needs in order to be able to evolve onward, to draw conclusions. . . .

Coronavirus: "cor" means "heart." In her book *New Days*[2] Christiane Beerlandt writes:

> Illnesses and ailments of the Heart and Blood Vessels tell us in these days: Thinking dominates the old world, served in the Drink of Desire — "Wanting to Have or Possess." Stress and agitation follow in the wake. As a consequence, the head is no longer FREE to serve the Heart — to receive, utilize or spread the beautiful messages of BEING, of LIFE.

Children very rarely fall ill from this coronavirus. So, every human being will do well to (re)discover, acknowledge and worship the spontaneous, playful, child-like aspect in oneself.

Which adult dares to behave like a happy, carefree child? Act the fool or the "maggot"? Horse around or wild out?

The child within you may be crowned king. The uninhibited child who can still play in nature, make discoveries, enjoy the simplest things.

Do you dare to show your true face? Are you prepared to show it? It's good to reflect about this — and about the symbolism of face masks — in times where they become increasingly visible in the streets, or even mandatory.

In life, do you feel like having your throat squeezed so tightly that you would almost suffocate? Is there something leaden, something that weighs on your shoulders? Emotions? Work? A relationship? . . . Does the sky seem heavy, dark, and threatening to you?

Do you feel like wearing a crown of thorns that stings and hurts so that the blood flows down your face, as it were? As if you have to carry a cross in this life, suffer a calvary? As if you are a prisoner dragging a leaden ball and chain?

Now liberate yourself COMPLETELY. You are ALLOWED. Breathe freely, live freely, enjoy freely. On the condition that this happens under the reign of Love, from out of the Heart.

No dogmas, no social, religious or other rules and norms that shackle you.

---

[2] This book hasn't yet been translated into English at the time of the publication of the present work.

Self-Love automatically leads to love for others.[3]

At the same time, you don't allow yourself to be parasitized, and you yourself don't sponge on others either.

Do you feel like an indecisive, despairing, somewhat helpless frog, looking up from below, with big eyes? "What will I do? Would I be able to . . .?"

Then realize that you can firmly and lovingly take the scepter of your life, like a trustful, wise Prince, wearing a strongly shining multicolored crown on your head. Rock-solidly present in yourself, your body of flesh and blood. Like in the fairy tale *The Twelve Gates of Prince Sirius*.[4]

Eggs, Easter eggs. . . . In her book *The Horn of Plenty*[5] Christiane Beerlandt devotes a chapter to the message of the egg, which says among other things:

> The human being who likes eggs seeks a haven of refuge in his own being. . . . The person who longs for an egg has the need to crawl deep Inside Himself — to completely turn inward and find there the Germ of his being. He will find himself anew within a sheltered, safe place. . . . He wishes for an indissoluble contact: with himself in the first place. . . . He wants to get closer to himself, his real Core. Closer, tighter, firmer, more solid. He wishes to forge a bond of unity that can no longer be undone by any force. . . .

Concentrate strongly within yourself. Direct yourself from out of this Essence. You are safe here; nothing can "destroy" you. . . . The human being takes care of life within himself. He will see to it that the child in his soul, his most sacred Life Essence, remains untouched.

Meanwhile, nature doesn't seem to worry about corona. Birds whistle and flutter merrily around. The sun offers light and warmth. Trees grow, blossom, bear fruits. Clouds float by and create magical sights. They give their rain. The wind caresses gently and brings fresh oxygen. The air became purer during the 2020 corona crisis.

Finally, this coronavirus would have "spilled over" from bats to humans. What message would bats want to give to the human being? About "not rushing by too fast"? About serene wisdom? About intuition, knowing without seeing? About false and true values? About the human being who is crowned Royal Human Being? About the most sacred child within the human being? In 2003 Christiane Beerlandt brought the message of the Bat to the human being, in her book *If Animals Could Talk . . .*[6]

In profound thankfulness to Christiane
Dr. Dirk Lippens
Lierde, 9 April 2020

---

[3] Read more about this on page 5 to 118 of the present book.
[4] This book hasn't yet been translated into English at the time of the publication of the present work.
[5] This book hasn't yet been translated into English at the time of the publication of the present work.
[6] This book hasn't yet been translated into English at the time of the publication of the present work. Other animals that could have played a role are the civet cat and the armadillo. And it's also interesting to listen to the messages of animals that would have been infected by humans: cat, dog, tiger, lion, mink. . . .

SARS

Severe Acute Respiratory Syndrome: pneumonia caused by the SARS coronavirus (SARS-CoV-1), with high fever, dry cough, shortness of breath

THE TEXT BELOW ALSO APPLIES TO SERIOUS CASES OF CoViD-19

●

Where does the SARS coronavirus find its breeding ground?

Not everyone who comes into contact with the SARS coronavirus gets infected. Not everyone infected with the SARS coronavirus dies. What is the ideal psycho-emotional breeding ground that the SARS coronavirus longs for? And, as a consequence, how can you do something about it on a psycho-emotional level — helping to chase the virus from your body?

Fundamental Origin

You feel like a dented car, as it were. Yearning for warm love, curled inward, contorted with pain and sorrows: as if you've just had to deal with a thrust in the stomach (mostly figuratively, at the level of your feelings . . .). You feel grabbed and painfully hurt. You've allowed this to "come in," into your being, prior to the virus penetrating inside your cells. The penetration of the virus is a consequence of the prior painful state.

You allow your joy to depend on experiences in the outside world. Time to go in search of the joy core inside yourself.

True self-love will lead to your not attracting situations in which you are hurt in your feelings.[7]

You are carrying heavy burdens , but it all seems like a vicious circle you can't get out of.

You experience yourself as a tree that has been beheaded; stripped of your crown and roots. Only the trunk remains, because "they" can use it. But in this way you can no longer draw any oxygen from the air. One takes you only for that which one needs from you: like one usually strips the white celery of its leaves and cuts the stalks into pieces to stew and eat.

Saturnal structures remain. The waving, cheerful Jupiter is being removed: no question about a happy, optimistic stream of thoughts.

You are not directed toward that which is Higher in yourself. You are not in contact with your inner root-core.

Life just seems boring and dull to you. You aren't exactly captivated. You're just standing there, like a little piggy that comes and looks indifferently and briefly at the humans.

There is some anger: "What on earth am I doing here?" You kick a couple of things in your vicinity, experiencing some kind of fundamental boredom and emptiness — as if you're mad at life itself.

Dark atmospheres that don't admit a glimpse of light. You're tired of it; you're standing there in a self-destructive manner.

---

[7] In this respect, more insights are given in the chapter about the Sixth Principle in the book *Alcyone — The Distorted Self-Image of the Human Being.* This work has not yet been translated into English at the publication of the present book.

You live on a not really conscious human level; perhaps this is similar to the brains of animals that don't really live CONSCIOUSLY, not experiencing the joy of life in a really conscious manner. In the same way, you experience the pointlessness of your existence. At a distance from your feelings, cut off from them.

"There's nothing *more* to life, isn't it?" That's what you ask, in doubt and despair. "Anyway, in this life there's nothing more than darkness, monotony. . . . Ah, what am I doing here on earth?" No laughter, but no tears either; a kind of emotional, affective death.

You put yourself in a structural, closed little circle, and then you experience yourself as a prisoner of your own system. A flattened brain that can't perceive any feeling anymore, so to speak. A dreary, flat, weary atmosphere: because you are closed off from the inner, living world of your feelings — from your inner, luminous source, your core.

Fundamental Solution

There is so much more in you! Immensely deep experiences and sensations of joy and bliss. Go in search of them; don't deny them to yourself. Solve those atmospheres of boredom and grayness in your presently limited world of experiences: first and foremost, by becoming aware of the fact that you've flattened yourself and have made yourself shrivel until you could no longer feel any happiness.

Discover the warmth of Love: first of all, love toward yourself, and then, while giving to yourself, love to others also. The 6 uncurls: lovingly giving. *In this flow full*

of love, the feeling of meaningfulness germinates: you will sense it. You can never develop enough love and emotional warmth in yourself; giving to yourself, giving to others.[8]

Vomit it all: your feelings of suppressed anger, dissatisfaction, the sadness hidden underneath. Come INTO DEEPLY FELT CONTACT with yourself. Ultimately, you end up at the center of yourself; you've emptied yourself. From out of this core, you can start anew — start all over. You've cleared yourself, you've brought all the concealed emotions to the surface: in this way you regain contact with yourself. You've discharged yourself from gloomy atmospheres.

You can start again at zero, but differently than before: Begin from the heart, while giving to yourself — in warmth and gratitude toward life. *Never again leave your INNER CORE OF FEELING.* Start from this warm central point of your being. Then, boredom won't occur anymore.

True love, true appreciation in yourself, dispels any form of dullness or tedium. The feeling, the feeling of love, now washes through your entire body; you experience a kind of joyful tingling in your body, your brain. Your compressed, flattened brain comes to life; it experiences light, joy, merriment, and meaningfulness: because of who you are, because of life in itself.

Transformation takes place; the body is turned inside out and has risen like a phoenix from its ashes. You now have become a truly LIVING human being: FEELING the joy, the meaningfulness of existence, of your "Being" in your body.

---

[8] In this respect, see The Sixth Land in *The Twelve Gates of Prince Sirius — The Quest for True Happiness.* This fairy tale by Christiane Beerlandt has not yet been translated into English at the publication of the present book.

FLU

(See also Infections, in General)[9]

Do you still believe in the system of "accidental contagion" by someone else? Know, then, that when you are not attuned to the vibration of the flu virus (see continuation of this text), you cannot be "infected" by it.

Unconsciously, you call up a time of rest for yourself. In *"working people"*: hectic, stressful life is so demanding on you. But also *"older people"* who are retired or bedridden, as well as *"babies"* and *"children"* at school or holiday camp, can develop a state of stress through inner tensions, feelings, anxious thoughts and experiences, etc.

It becomes too much for you, as does the busyness around you; you'd like to be peacefully alone for a little while — a flu will permit this. You throw out the anchor.

The outer world seems threatening to you; you wish to withdraw into a safe shell. You feel like a slave in a social, or other, system; your personal feelings are not allowed to count — tension, frustrations, sadness. The outbreak of flu hinders more serious illnesses from developing themselves. (Just allow a cold, fever, or flu to come through, and don't suppress it. However, do use medicine when things get out of hand and the fundamental cause cannot be solved in the now moment.)

Flu, therefore, is like a pair of tongs which seize you and simultaneously offer protection. That is what you prefer to look for: a safe shelter, rest.

Accumulated energies (emotions, thoughts, creativity) seek a way out.

Flu is often an indication that you are unsure and afraid; "Am I doing it right?" You're perhaps afraid to take total responsibility regarding a certain task. You're afraid of reprimand; fear of failure. Possibly you are overburdened. You fiercely use your elbows, but you fear that it's not all going to work out. You feel like a SLAVE.

Feelings of oppression, insecurity, and anxiety, not trusting in your own Basis: this all breaks down your immunity.[10]

Are you allowing yourself to be influenced too much by your surroundings? Do you refuse to live autonomously, "from out of yourself"?

Live YOURSELF, not trained like a circus animal. Clearly determine your limits, full of self-confidence!

Experience your inner powers, your immune system, the cheerfulness and warmth in your original nature. Feel welcome among people, dare to enjoy; know yourself to be safe in your Living self, and don't let yourself be rushed by anything or anyone! Becoming infected only happens if you unconsciously ask for it (to bring about changes in yourself); you are naturally immune.

Don't allow yourself to be influenced by negativity in your surroundings: be faithful to yourself.

You do accomplish your tasks, that's true — balancing, in equilibrium, like a hen above its eggs, giving as much to the left as to the right — but you stagnate in this so-called perfect state. Are you a machine, a controllable robot? You surely are not, are you? Why let yourself be like a geometrically perfect model — not being someone who is *really* LIVING, from out of your *original NATURE*? You needn't be "polished," "still," "perfect."

---

[9] See the book *The Key to Self-Liberation.*
[10] See the chapter: Immune Deficiency Diseases (in *The Key to Self-Liberation*).

Come to life, being open, direct, spontaneous, continuously developing yourself! Break out of those habits, that self-built structural column; quit the Old.

Renewal! Breathing new life into yourself. You as YOU — not as a mere number, a little monkey, just a drop in the sea of people. No longer camouflage yourself by immersing yourself in a work, an attitude, a tradition, a family structure, or whatever. *Give yourself a **face** — unique and authentic. You as You. Allow **evolution** and spontaneous Growth to set in. Do not make anything fixed, immutable — including yourself. Or are you like a box of building blocks, where the blocks can be stacked gradually, and where only the matching block is allowed on top?* You are not like that, are you? You are a human being who will do well to be open to innovations and unexpected turns, to adaptations and natural versatility. Your NATURE calls you! Have you hidden it under the building block structure for too long? *Evolution is required; thawing, suppleness toward your own nature.* You surely are not a static structural device, are you?

You will do well to go ahead with firm steps, walking in the direction of infinity. Don't put a stop to yourself, to life, but go onward with vigorous, dynamic strides. No longer stand still in evolution; don't stagnate in old habits. *Don't paralyze yourself in a suffocating, tidily balanced "system" in which "the human being" has got lost! BREAK open. Go out. Break out of your self-designed prison structure.* FEEL the primal power in your arms, your legs. Connect to the true life core that is in you.

Feel how the fire of life flows through your members in a healthy way; take pleasure in this sensation. You, supple and flexible, vigorously going onward, you open yourself up to your BECOM-

ING, your true birth, dynamic and never-ending. You are free now; you can breathe for yourself, from out of yourself. You show who you are; you've given yourself a character, a true face. You now fully ACKNOWLEDGE your being, your uniqueness. You no longer hide behind a mountain of paper work, a series of excuses, glasses of beer, all kinds of hobbies, an illness, powerlessness, or whatever. *Yes: YOU are there . . . underneath all of this, behind all of this. Come and show yourself. FEEL who you ARE! Then live from out of, and according to, this genuine sensitive being of your "I"!*

●

The Why of Influenza at Global Level

●

You are infected with an influenza virus and it makes you ill, and: WHY there are always appearing new and more serious variants of the influenza virus, causing an epidemic or even a pandemic

●

Fundamental Origin

In fact, life asks for **a "rescue operation" of the human being and humanity** by making the virus appear and penetrate human beings. The aim is that the human being would become aware that he can no longer live in an unconscious manner, in a kind of self-destructive way, as he has done so far.

Ultimately, Life wants to establish itself definitively in the human being, in physical immortality. It sends its death's advocate (so-called dangerous viruses), as it were, so that the human being would react against it: by realizing that it is not the virus, illness, death, that is master over him — but that The Human Being himself is Master over his life and has everything in him to conquer this viral illness, death, forever.

Becoming aware, insight into life and death, and the realization that death is not ineluctable: the influenza virus gives a foretaste of this. **A new era is dawning. The human being who has become Aware will now have to Choose Life or Death and live accordingly.**

Not every human being gets infected by a virus; not every person who has been in contact with the influenza virus becomes ill: he remains healthy because the breeding ground for the virus is not present in him. This breeding ground lies underneath the surface — on a psychological-emotional level, in the convictions and thought patterns according to which the human being lives.

Stepping out of the herd mentality pattern. Then, initially as a "modest human," highly unique and individual, he will grow into an indestructible, good-hearted Human Being, strong in belief, who takes the reins over his life.

Also see the text: Immune Deficiency Diseases (in *The Key to Self-Liberation*).

●

Why does the Influenza Virus enter your body and give a wake-up call?

Like a giant pumpkin[11] with claws, you grab at the earth: the fruit, fully loaded with potentialities, desires the earth; it absolutely wants to . . . it will not and it shall not unhook its paws from the piece of earth it is sitting on — like a crab, instinctively. On earth is where you want to be, and this can't be taken away from you. Desiring to grab hold of . . . . Basically, this self-preservation instinct is a very positive thing; at the same time, however, you will also have to connect yourself to the vibration of BEING — this means abstaining from GRABBING (be it in thought or deed), from WANTING TO HAVE OR POSSESS. After all, this grabbing lies in the extension of death.

Yes, this illness asks you to let go; to come home to your "I," your BEING. Come to the understanding that those primordial pumpkin powers inside you now ask for a Transformation, a conversion of instinctive energies into conscious creational powers.

Starting to live and act differently; putting an end to the habitual way of life from the past (including even **unconscious** thoughts, expectations . . . such as in babies, people growing demented, etc.).

For instance: To BE, to Live as an "I" — instead of wanting to grab or possess things or people, accompanied by impatience and dissatisfaction, or desire to achieve, ambition, wanting to be approved by others, or anger because one doesn't give you what you want to obtain, etc., etc. To utilize *true* creation powers — instead of losing yourself in "the spirit," drugs, alcohol, empty sex (for self-gratification or gratification of someone else), superficial activities, games, watching tv for hours and hours, nagging and gossiping, etc. In sum, this illness asks you to BE on earth in a CONSCIOUS and LOVINGLY GIVING manner.

Unconsciously you are searching for a channel to drain away your feelings. It's like a man who looks down from high a-

---

[11] See the deeper symbolic meaning of the Pumpkin in *The Horn of Plenty*. This work has not yet been translated into English at the publication of the present book.

bove the earth's surface while his urine seeks the metal tube of the urinal in order to let his water flow through it. In this way he liberates himself; however, this doesn't alter the fact that he dwells very far away, high above the Earth, his head way up in the sky, distant.

The influenza virus — and its possible companion, fever[12] — are like a prod; they offer the human being an opportunity to connect with the earthly. The influenza virus can penetrate cells because, among other things, there is a distance between the human being and himself, his content, his feelings, his real deep nature, his primal powers, his potential transformational energy.

Continuously wanting to let go, discharge; and in itself, this outlet is a good thing: urine, "water" — symbolic of pent-up or unexpressed feelings, suppressed creativity; "oil" — meaning that one hasn't consciously exploited one's energies; pus — representing the fact that one sees life as dark and heavy; "mud"; emotions dark as ink; stress; etc., etc.: anything that needs to drain off to the earth, running fluidly. Wanting to dispose of dirt stored in the body, via the kidneys for instance. One cleanses oneself in this way: by allowing a loose flow. Before pouring new oil into a car, one first drains away old, impure, used oil residues. Let it all run out. It is required to achieve absolute purity.

Like an animal that opens its mouth very wide in order to receive that which comes flying in; to catch and consume it, eagerly but passively. It waits patiently and, in so doing, there is no active leap forward. Like a little bird that waits and knows for sure that food will be brought by its moth-

er; this symbolizes the unconscious instinct of trust in the primal womb. One does not really undertake anything, act as an "I." One lets oneself droop, or the human being allows himself to "be lived" by others, or, simply, he lives in unconsciousness: the virus can easily enter.

The white toilet bowl overflows, a large wide stream brims over, but it turns out to be pure water now: the overspill of water flows over the edge toward the earth without stopping, as it were.

You put your forearm[13] crosswise on the strings of a violin or a guitar, impeding . . . prohibitive, preventing any sound to pour out of the sound box. You put a strong pressure on it; it's as if you say: "No, this is not allowed." In this case, it's about a severity toward yourself: as if you prevent your talents, your beautiful feelings, your golden sounds, from externalizing themselves.

The upper part of the body, shoulders, upper arms, are rather tightened, tensely contracted, the shoulders and the head trembling with chill, so it seems: as if you want to lay an egg but can't get it out.

Somewhat wide-eyed with fear, not getting a clear view of, nor a grip on, the lower part of your body: it looks like you aren't master of your totality, your entire physical being, your life's course. You don't succeed in managing things anymore. "Help, what will I do?" You seem to be under electric stress, as it were. High voltage.

At the same time, one would say that you are absent — your "I," who is supposed to be at the head of your Life, doesn't seem to be there.

---

[12] See the underlying meaning of fever in the relevant section of *The Key to Self-Liberation*.
[13] See the general symbolism of the forearm in the relevant section of *The Key to Self-Liberation*.

Fundamental Solution

Allow your basis, your body, your entire being to unfold on the earth's surface. As if your living Self-Essence asks you to *let yourself drop, completely and widely, on the earth, so that "the spirit" wouldn't have a grip on you anymore.* "The spirit" is in the first place your own spirit, of course: the head, thinking, being in the mind — instead of being one with the earth, your body, your feeling. When there's too great a distance between spirit and earth, then put an end to this: nestle down, spread yourself on the earth like in a rounded form. Nothing can leave this earth anymore — not one part of yourself. An Eternal Alliance with the earth.

It's like the alpine horn whose reverb hole descends to earth, allowing its deep bass sound to stream out from there into the entire world. From out of the blowing mouth, the pipe, through which the sound flows, first searches for the earth down there, and then that magnificent sound spreads *tangibly*.

It is clear: do not speak or express yourself from the head, from ethereal spheres, from out of some kind of absence from your physical, earthly being — but from the heart, the center of your belly, of your being. FEEL! Feel and LIVE from out of your earthly body. Do not live from the head and thoughts.

First sink lovingly into yourself — toward the bottom of yourself, of the earth. You now are one with your body, having entirely descended into yourself. You aren't away from the earthly being-here-and-now anymore, in no respect whatsoever.

Ultimately, this is a prerequisite for developing in you that which the Source of Life finally intends for the Human Being — or that which your absolutely unique Self-Essence intends for you: the evolution toward physical immortality. You can get it started now. The human being doesn't have to suffer, die, bid farewell to beloved friends because of physical death; once the human being imposed this limitation on himself. The time has come for the human being to see how he can turn this around. . . .[14]

But everyone is free to choose their own path.

•

Penetration of a Virus

It should come as no surprise that, for instance, in 2003[15] an aggressive virus struck and immobilized many people in my country, Belgium. A reader let me know that he hadn't been that sick for years, despite the fact that he tried so hard to do all the right things for his physical and mental well-being.

Then I looked at **the purpose** of that virus. And actually this goes for all kinds of viruses:

- You, as a human being, should realize more strongly who you are, and THAT you are; that you exist as an "I"; and that you are able to establish yourself even more powerfully as an "I."

- This presupposes that you make undesirable things harmlessly glance off you: everything that threatens to enter by devious ways and doesn't really be-

---

[14] Read more about this in *New Days,* as well as in other books by the same author. This work has not yet been translated into English at the publication of the present book.
[15] Numerologically, 2003 represents the frequency of working on one's autonomy and immunity.

long with you. Don't pay attention to the negative that would like to come and disturb your warm, positive energy field.

- Self-rejection should be eliminated on every level. Rejecting yourself can happen in different ways: Why aren't you satisfied with yourself? Is it the content of who you are that displeases you? Is it your external appearance? Your "performances"? (Desiring to achieve certain "performances" may not correspond to living on the wavelength of True Life.) Are you afraid that others would consider you ugly or negative? Afraid of being not good enough? Of being not strong enough? Are you so demanding on yourself?

- This virus was a TEST. It helps make you stronger, both inwardly and physically. Taken down by a virus? In bed for a week? Vomiting? You are being compelled to go in search of yourself, very deeply, and conduct a thorough self-examination. What makes you dissatisfied with yourself? What is it in you that nauseates you?[16] Do you put demands on yourself that you cannot meet?

Begin to love yourself UNCONDITIONALLY. Your TRUE, ORIGINAL "I" is not hard and demanding, is not small or scared, on the contrary! A purification is required; a rediscovery of your inconceivably strong, loving, authentic "I."

Everything you regret — try to correct it where this is necessary.

Turn toward yourself and examine in what respect you feel yourself to be a failure — in which regard you approach yourself in a destructive way (albeit slightly). Because in the same way — through this entrance door — the virus can approach you in a destructive manner.

Love. Gentleness. Self-acknowledgement. Not wanting to satisfy this or that rule or value.

Just be yourself as you are. Don't run yourself down, in any respect; correct yourself where necessary. Don't work your body to death.

With this flu-like virus, some people are particularly troubled by a sore throat, others have intestinal problems, suffer from vomiting, coughing, painful joints, ...[17] Your weakest spot is now brought to the surface and shown. Yes, via the entry of the virus, your soul core now shows you exactly where to work on yourself the most: see the corresponding chapters in this book and *The Key to Self-Liberation*.

•

Two days later, I received a message from the same reader: **the mirror** of his car had been shattered after hitting another car.

Why do there have to be mirrors? Of course, car mirrors are essential for safety. But what about all the mirrors that we have in our houses? What if, for once, we all undertook to live without mirrors? Just living from deep within — from the heart, according to what we *feel* deep inside? The reader concerned had just said to his partner: "Look how old I'm getting. Balding, full of wrinkles. . . ." So what does that matter? It's really of no importance whatsoever.

Wrinkles are a sign of getting on in years healthily and solidly; they are not a

---

[16] See the psycho-emotional origins of nausea and vomiting in *The Key to Self-Liberation*.
[17] If necessary, see the chapters about the intestines, diarrhea, intestinal cramps, the throat, coughing, the joints, etc., in *The Key to Self-Liberation*.

sign of decline. They indicate, among other things, that deep-lying experiences are being lived, but they have NOTHING to do with illness or death. The same goes for balding.

That's also what the virus tells you: Why be so concerned with your external appearance? Why ask yourself the question: "How do I look like?" That's of no significance at all, isn't it? When you feel good from the inside, when you ARE yourself in your body, as you are — with or without skin discolorations or wrinkles, with or without hair or little warts, plump or thin, tall or small — then what does this matter in the eyes of Life? True beauty goes hand in hand with GOODNESS, and you can see that in the body. It has nothing to do with sham beauty and fashion trends.

An aggressive flu-like virus, coronavirus, etc.? Don't be afraid but do what you have to do. Just like every human being, you need to check inside yourself and ask if there's something in you that you don't like — that you condemn, consider in a destructive or aggressive way (as aggressive as the "eyes" of the virus).

Also, live according to the conviction that you are stronger than any so-called enemy from the outside. When you live in Love, then the power in your being is so immense, gentle, and loving, that any aggressive, intruding virus will just bounce off harmlessly. Strongly believe in yourself. Know that you are a good person. And that you are no VICTIM of evil as long as you cherish yourself within the fence of Love.

Do light bulbs in your house blow frequently and loudly? Then reflect about this: Is there too much hardness in your deeds or thoughts? Do you condemn yourself or others? Do you get tensed up by things that happen? Do you harden? Then you shouldn't be surprised that there's an electricity problem.[18]

Listen to your heart; don't lose yourself into what you are doing, into your work, into what's happening around you. Stay very closely involved with yourself. Solve the last remnants. Go deeper into yourself.

At any moment, give yourself the chance to do what you feel you have to do. Let go immediately when you feel, "I am carrying too heavy a burden, I continue working although I feel I have to stop."

Listen to that language. Lovingly become master of your existence. So don't at all feel like a victim. Be convinced that any aggressive virus can stay out — that at the very most it may drop by for a little while and then leave immediately — provided you have understood its message and don't oppose resistance to necessary changes you have to make.

What about people who are severely struck by the aggressive virus?

You are unable to "do" anything anymore. You are stuck in bed. You are in pain. Everything is knocked out of your hands, so to say, in order for you to arrive at the ESSENCE of your "I." No more escape route.

Come close to yourself, very lovingly. Don't be angry but try to understand. Trust that your body will defend itself adequately. Believe and trust that you will get through. It will be so.

---

[18] The psychological correspondence of a light bulb that blows is explained in *The Signal Book*. This book hasn't yet been translated into English at the publication of the present work.

Of course you can take medicine or herbs, as long as you don't use them only as a SUBSTITUTE for the *real* solution.

So, let remedies from the outside and personal growth go together. Ask yourself, "Why?" Are you still so far away from your *true* core? So far away from this warm love for yourself? In anxiety, "Who am I? Am I nothing but a . . .?"

In order that you would realize: "I am a human being. Not 'just' a human being, but A Human Being who is now asked to come very, very close to himself — in an intense, loving union — and to shed every old, false value."

Abandon every judgment, every worth assessment, with regard to yourself and others.

Start to live from the inside out, a hundred percent. Not: "How do I look like?" But: "How do I feel? Will I finally begin to completely live from within outward, honestly from the heart? What others say or think about me plays no role at all, isn't that true?"

The deepest discovery of the "I." Being happy and satisfied, yes, healthily proud about this "I."

No judgment whatsoever toward others, but a complete letting go and understanding.

You should now be occupied with yourself. You are ill. You can't do anything else but to be involved with yourself: dive into your own depths. Come home to yourself, deep down in your warm heart, your bone marrow. Let go: empty your head. Go in search of what you feel inside: feel yourself, sense yourself.

And then, purpose to live in a *giving* way: give to yourself, give to others.

But you never run past YOURSELF again. Should you feel, even in the slightest way, that you are falling back in that pattern, then bring yourself back "inside"; turn your eyes inward and stay on in the deepest house of your "I." The

virus compels you to get yourself back inside your own "I," your own body, time and again.

In this period of time, this is necessary and beneficial for people who are plagued with a flu-like virus, coronavirus, etc. Finally, they can emerge strengthened, grown, and purified.

And when these steps are taken properly, the human being stands stronger against any next aggressive virus attack. Because no matter what virus is knocking at the door, the Human Being has found himself back — more strongly and deeply — and Virus number X will now have a very hard time getting in.

Again, the human being is one step ahead.

Therefore, don't consider a viral infection as negative, but as a victory — often it is a whole step forward. Though, of course, this doesn't have to happen.

Trust your Nature. Trust your signals. And take the necessary steps. Turn your body into a "House of Delight"!

•

About Air and Airways
Open yourself up.
Surrender to Life, to your
own vast Being

In order that no germ, no virus can have a negative impact on your airways.

The respiratory tract symbolizes, on the one hand, breathing in: breathing in life, in an unlimited way. Providing your body enthusiastically and happily with life oxygen.

On the other hand, breathing out: discharging everything that no longer needs to be present in you, including your worries, tensions, thoughts that prevent you from "being."

The human being who "thinks" with Descartes, "Je pense, donc je suis" — "I think, therefore I am" — is not in deeply felt contact with the profound inner knowing. He wants to reason and think about everything and doesn't dare to build upon his capacity to *feel* into his depths — trusting inner knowledge. He probably wouldn't even understand what we're talking about here.

Still, *every* human being on earth has the possibility to open wide the "crown" of his head — to connect with an inner knowing, to feel and intuitively know with heart and brain, with his entire being.

The only thing is that he then needs to stop his thinking for a moment — turning inward, coming very close to himself, letting go of everything outside himself, and learning to feel and sense. He will intuit knowledge that can barely be comprehended or rendered by thinking.

It's about the melting pot, the point of fusion, of all the riches that are present in a human being — opulent elements which are difficult to name: wisdom, feeling, intuition, a kind of wise thinking power that doesn't mean merely "thinking."

The deeper knowing, the deeper feeling.

Your airways ask you to establish contact with yourself: **to go *very* deep into your own being and to experience there that Unlimitedness**.

Put a stop to exaggerated thinking or "false emotionality." You think with anger, you think with sadness . . . whereas your being is actually Joy, feeling joy, knowing joy.

The essential "I" that you are has strayed away when your "I" gets lost into the mere thinking — into the emotional that deviates from a healthy train of thought, from genuine deeper knowing, from feelings experienced in purity.

A healthy emotional release is a very good thing when needed; however, as soon as you begin to wallow in a kind of emotionality that doesn't serve life, this only lowers you (for example, pity, feelings of guilt, etc.).

Sympathy and *understanding* are good but don't let yourself be dragged down into a short-sighted vision. If you want to help the world, the wisest thing to do is to stay on the shore or on the Bridge.

Know that everyone creates their own life, consciously or unconsciously; understand this principle. Pass on your knowledge when asked for it: better this than to jump also into the deep water and drown.

So create your life; adjust your course where necessary. Above all, experience yourself deeply, *feel* into your depths; feel into the depths of life.

Don't lose yourself in rarefied heights, nor in narrow-minded or emotional thinking and pondering.

Don't suffocate yourself with these things; don't suffocate yourself by not giving your "I" all **Space** it deserves. Don't block or corner yourself by grabbing or grasping — by not living on an autonomous basis.

Free your mind, your head from spinning thoughts and emotions. Turn toward the joyful emotion that is called "the flow of life." Relax regularly when you feel that you are running through life in a way that is too tense.

Come home to yourself. Open yourself up. Don't confine yourself in any way.

Know that eventually, truth always prevails.

Don't disrespect others' borders; don't let others transgress your borders. You will do well to take care of your piece of open green pasture; take up your responsibility.

Don't oblige yourself or others; no pressure. Because airways love to feel freedom. Don't coerce yourself. Carry yourself into the free space of life.

ENJOY. Play. Open your lungs. Reach with your hands to the farthest horizons of happiness without wanting to grab them.

Let go, throw the dead weight of the past overboard. Don't linger in anger or resentment. Open yourself up completely.

BREATHE FREELY AND BLISSFULLY AS "I"-THE-HUMAN-BEING.

Your airways want to feel the free life, looking out on an infinite, joyful perspective.

And is there still sadness, anxiety, anger, or whatever other emotion[19] present in you? Take a good look at them and solve them, so that you empty yourself of things that you would drown in.

Then bring yourself to dry land — or even better, purify the water inside yourself, filter it, while still enjoying a delicious swim in the pure, cleansing life-water.

In this way, you also chase away all viruses that could have an impact on the respiratory system.

AUTISM

Fundamental Origin and Solution

An autistic person believes too little in himself, *condemning* himself to failure.

He comes into life with a feeling of being shut out, of being a marginal person, a beggar, an unrecognized artist who lives in an attic somewhere.

Nevertheless, he is full of ambitions, talents — but the feeling of incapability and the fear of being *hurt,* cast out, or devoured by others, causes him to *shut himself out.* From the urge to protect himself he builds a strong wall around his personality.

Inwardly, he is *fastidious, critical.* In his thinking patterns, he develops himself into a perfectionist; in his thoughts he is always busy realizing his ambitions, small as they might be.

But he doesn't get anywhere with this perfectionism regarding himself, certainly not when he already feels himself to be so incapable: "I know I can't do it." When it comes to these *critical standards* he places on himself, he fails completely: "I am horribly bad and not worthy to really live fully."

Indeed, others might only reinforce this. He locks himself behind high walls. In this way, he gets the *attention* he so longs for, and does so without being condemned for his bad aspects — for is he not sick and unreachable?

By being a mirror for the suppressed problems of the parents, the child can allow the parents to evolve.

The parents can allow the child to evolve by not trying to flee from the psychological situation, but by resolving it in

---

[19] Read more about this on page 5 to 118 of the present book, as well as the chapter Emotions, in *The Key to Self-Liberation*.

themselves. The *fears,* the conviction, that they, themselves, don't *meet certain requirements* in order to be good human beings. . . . The fear that the world is, in fact, an unsafe place in which to exist. . . . All the above-mentioned causes also need to be considered introspectively by the parents (*self-criticism, self-demolition,* etc.).

Hospitality, warmth, security: for yourself, for others!

*Anxieties are the reason a child doesn't dare to **truly** come out of his shell until everything is safe. At that moment, it is best that one let him come out by himself. An attempt by the autistic person to communicate — even if, for instance, it is only asking for a cookie when he has not had solid food for far too long. The turtle only shows its head when it intuitively feels it will be safe, that people will not consider it an ugly worthless being and crush it.*

Because after all he doesn't approve of himself, he is sensitive to judgment and criticism from the outside, and he hides.

It is therefore of absolute importance that the autistic person can develop his special talents without hindrance or criticism from the outside. In this way, he can start to eliminate self-criticism and self-destruction. Without those who raise him having to go along in a kind of power-game that is being set up.

Indeed, autistic persons are often "specially gifted" in one area or another, but question their own worth too critically, even break themselves down.

They give themselves, and also their surroundings, this lesson of life: *everyone may and must experience his own unique Nature without attaching "norms, demands, or expectations" to human development.* There happen to be several ways to be "gifted" that our Western society does not understand (yet).

It is of extreme importance for the autistic person to know that — because of his unique Nature — he is "welcome and accepted." Being allowed to FREELY be himself, and yet still be "safe": still, first of all, he will have to GIVE this to himself . . . and should not expect anything from others.

Thus, he can respect his own Worthiness; thus, the "static" he has built up with regard to his own "I" — in a critical, disparaging, condemnatory way — can be resolved.

Only if he has esteem for, and awareness of his Worthy "I" can he come, without fear, into Contact with others.

To the person who experiences himself as autistic, we would like to say:

You stab yourself, your "I," inwards, as it were, as if Mars sticks his arrow into your body. As if it's about a deep-seated pain in the root of your tooth.

Of course, you hurt yourself in a form of *self-destruction,* not loving yourself enough or not at all; hard and critical, painfully pushing yourself down, *suppressing yourself,* holding yourself under water, *refusing* yourself to exist in peace, joy, cheerfulness and painlessness. You want to *punish* yourself, as it were, with all the sins of the world, and you will "do penance for it."

This conviction lives in you! Why? It has no single true reason; *only you can judge yourself: "Am I a good or a bad human being?"*

Decide that you are a good human being and live accordingly; offer yourself that which is most beautiful, most wonderful, most happy in life!

Descend that dark staircase. Were you fleeing? Then come back, come back down!

Only you can make yourself appear or disappear. Only you are the one who punishes yourself . . . and do so without cause! *There's no evil in you, you are not bad, life is not bad.*

Or do you really want to make yourself believe this, so that you have no reason to come to life, to rise above water? You are not a coward are you?

Or do you want to play a *power game* with your surroundings, *asking for attention* in a certain way, even if it is by keeping yourself hidden? Then it's impossible for you to think yourself "good."

So, choose to Live, you as a wonderful "I" . . . or choose to remain dwelling in dark cellars of power and self-destruction and playing games with your surroundings.

*Life, your Heart, begs YOU to bring YOURSELF toward **true** Life, in honest communication with others.*

This can only happen when first you come into warm, heartfelt contact with yourself, when you no longer crawl away from Life again and again. But the choice, of course, is up to you!

Do you want to keep yourself unhappy, punish yourself, not live? Or do you want to offer yourself life, make yourself happy?

Listen well for once to what your inner heart asks of you. And then you will hear from your heart that "you are not a bad person, that you have to stop hiding yourself and in a condemning way pulling yourself down" . . . and that it has become time *that YOU — and no one else — bring YOURSELF to life.* Life will be thankful to you!

Now call yourself to order, take yourself RESOLUTELY by the shoulders and say to yourself: "What do you want, what are you actually going to do now, what are you going to make of your life? Do you want to die or do you want to live? Do you want to flee or are you going to take yourself by the hand and make something wonderfully beautiful of your existence? The choice is yours!"

Stand up, go onward and become master over your feelings with strong, assertive forces, with a primal life force that is in you; feelings and negative thoughts never have to run away with you.

Make a break with dark, negative convictions. Take hold of yourself and make something beautiful of your life. It is up to you — that CHOICE of true "life"!!

Live from out of your Heart; believe in yourself, in your goodness. Someone else won't do this for you. What will you do?

CARSICKNESS

Fundamental Origin

In daily life you feel oppressed, wedged in an iron structure (like the structure of a car); you are too cold and too hard with yourself. Warm feelings of love cannot sufficiently flow in your heart; perhaps you feel suffocated under strong, authoritarian domination.

However, this severe authority lives within yourself in the first place. Anxiety, lack of self-confidence, anger because of your feelings of "being stuck."

Emotions weigh heavily on you; you lack insight into "how to deal with your feeling life." You ache (unconsciously) for self-liberation, for freedom.

Fundamental Solution

Therefore, allow your own feelings to blossom in warmth! Place the sun-center inside you; it's no use to resist an authority, because the true problem is your inability to achieve self-realization. Warm yourself; dare to EXPRESS yourself fully so that anxieties, coldness, and self-entrapment disappear. You are becoming carsick because you don't yet really live from out of your self-aware "I," because you don't yet know yourself to be really secure and protected in your deepest

Self, because you feel as if someone has seized you by the wrists, even if this needn't be the case in reality.

You, yourself, need to release yourself from your inner prison. Arrive at joyous self-expression. Allow the content of your being to flow freely. You no longer feel imprisoned now. Sing, talk, laugh, express what you feel . . . take up your space. As a result, you will also attract liberating situations in the outer world. (For instance, a harsh teacher disappears, there's no constraint or "having to" anymore, etc.)

CELIAC DISEASE

intolerance or allergy to gluten, which may cause damage to the wall of the small intestine

---

Fundamental Origin

You don't see a way out (anymore); you blame it perhaps on certain things which you have experienced, but the fundamental cause lies in the deep-seated sadness (with which you were born) which now asks to be cleaned up: by looking at it, by also "experiencing" your feelings in order to finally come to Insight and a Solution.

Initially, it seems as if your eyes are veiled; it seems as if you can't right away come in loving, peaceful contact with yourself as "a human being existing on earth." No longer hide behind a face that doesn't show anything, but tell about it — how you feel, how you are doing — don't keep walking around with it, but for once get it all out if need be. Leave your coat on the coat hanger — for you don't have to run away, again and again, when you feel a deep truth will be touched. Don't flee, don't hide. Don't escape from your deeper feelings, even if it's about sad-

ness and fear. Don't flee from any pure confrontation with yourself — what you feel deep inside — even if this is sometimes through contact with others. Look at it, experience your feelings, and see: it all becomes clearer and better! Honest confrontation with yourself, with your deepest feelings, and as a result things can clear up in the contact with yourself, with certain other people.

You feel damaged, as it were; your brain hurts from the gloominess, the anxiety, and the pain, possibly in remembrance of the Past. An original sadness because you actually feel rejected from the primal womb . . . because you make your love and happiness dependent on things and people outside yourself.

Come to acknowledge yourself, welcome yourself lovingly. This is the only way to solve a kind of primal sadness. Stop denying the greatness in yourself. Know that you attract every situation in life yourself, be it unconsciously: you have brought yourself to earth now in order to get to know *true* Life and *true* Joy!

Therefore, don't remain stuck in the obscure primal spheres "where it was so much better." That, it is not. You only fool yourself with it, because you don't succeed in comforting yourself, welcoming yourself in a warm way. Experience your sadness . . . but finally choose Joy.

You have to DO something, and you know it; you can't keep running in place. In order to arrive at a delightful experience of yourself as an earthly "I," start with feeling yourself, expressing yourself, in an honest way — with giving up your Old Image, stepping out of the Old Straitjacket and offering yourself absolute Freedom to Live, doing what you feel you have to do, going where you feel you have to go at any moment of the day. Don't cling to something or someone, but go onward! Very deeply, and truly, from out of your Content! Only in this way can you make a breach in your being where it is necessary.

Fundamental Solution

Don't persist in the same old vicious circle, but now make a step forward. If necessary break open a door, bike through the streets — so to speak — loudly ringing your bicycle bell, making lots of noise. EXPRESS YOURSELF.

Allow energies of truth, feelings, to flow freely through your being so that you might start to realize that life on earth means "Joy" in your greatest self and not sadness.

You don't have to blindfold your eyes; you may completely be yourself! Show YOUR worthiness and your "maturity," your "fullness," and no longer put yourself down. Hang your laundry out to dry and let the old dirt and emotions drip out.

Turn deeply inward into your heart and no longer allow yourself to be overpowered by emotions from the far and vague past, when you didn't really exist as "I." You are you in the NOW. Come closer to yourself and take yourself joyfully in! Yes, you belong completely: stop closing yourself out! In this way, sadness makes space for joy and chilliness for warmth. Yes, a warm welcome for yourself; now you see things in an optimistic perspective; your eyes light up! You no longer want to flee from yourself, from earthly existence, because now you know that you have everything in hand: your joy and your sadness. In a joyful way, you say "yes" to yourself, to your body, to your existence on earth as "I"; you no longer see yourself and life as an inevitably sad happening, but you come fully to the realization that you truly belong, that Life on earth in your body means Joy: an acknowledgement of your total "I," a rehabilitation, a warm welcome, no longer fleeing from your true content, from the warm joy in your heart.

Throwing off an old sore and surrendering to Life, which wants to fully flow through you, like a large river in its riverbed: also literally, in your digestive organs, in your intestines. Warmly come home to yourself and no longer consider yourself as a "sad" happening; arrive at an honest Alliance with yourself, your body, life. Enjoy yourself, your body, take pleasure in the contact with your true content, in the contact with others. Yes, you come completely home to yourself. You eliminate every anxiety, every old sadness: because you, yourself, now create your experience of Joy from the Heart. You no longer allow yourself to "be lived": you take the reins over your life in your hands!

The choice has been made.

INTESTINAL CANCER

Intestinal Cancer, in General

Fundamental Origin

Deep, vague anxieties. . . . You don't know where they come from, but you think you are sliding away into a deep, dark hole. You have the impression that you are at the mercy of a dizzying, turning Wheel, which you can't do anything about. You don't direct your life *yourself.* Fear of being gone, of being toppled, of losing all control — powerlessness.

You hold on to something, but at the same time you'd like to throw it away. "Help! My horse is bolting, and I can't get hold of the reins. . . ." Afraid of your deepest Self, of your emotions, of your natural feelings: you keep yourself hidden under a metal structure.

●

As if your pulmonary membrane reacts in a pink-red manner, with sadness. You don't see a way out anymore. You are in pain. A cough that kind of tears you up inside would like to break through, but you stammer and shrink together; you don't really say what the bottom line is all about. It's like the sorrow about losing a loved one, a loved thing. Purple-rose-pink, those are the colors that characterize your personal atmosphere. In your feelings, you are already sounding the death bell, be it unconsciously; but you don't realize that you can choose the path of your resurgence. It all depends on your inner choice: Do you still want to be here? Or can you no longer see the sense in things? You don't express that which is deepest. . . .

A sensitive person, sensitive membranes in your intestinal system, in all the inner walls of your body. A character of gold, but no one knows if you *really* exist or if you are in the spiritual spheres. *Where* are you really? Who *are* you? Do you live hidden in a role, a function? Where is your strong, *true* "I"? Where are those treasures of gold hidden?

The causes lie deep inside you, like the lees in a bottle of red wine. Yes, the symbolism of red wine[20] asks you to come full-bloodedly inside yourself, your body; to not flee to spiritual spheres, to spheres in which you are no longer present IN yourself. There may be external appearances, an image, a job, a joke, but where is your *true* "I AM"? We are not seeing it yet.

As if no knife can sharpen you: that's how blunt you have been (or still are) with yourself, and possibly also with your close friends. Why such gruffness? Why chase the sweet sounds, love itself, to the distant abysses?

Fragile, breakable; brittle bones like those of a nearly departed human being,

but you don't care about it; you feel too cold in life anyway. Others can do with you all they want, but if you yourself do not want to come to life, then everything is of no avail.

How many times did you ask yourself, "Why am I here? What am I doing here? How could there be anything worthwhile to be found here on earth?" You are not *really* here. The true meaning of existence escapes you. Dissatisfaction or disappointment about yourself or a situation you are in right now, do the rest.
You will have to choose! Choose in favor of "I LIVE MEANINGFULLY IN MY BEING," or in favor of "It all makes no sense; is life only this?" The consequences of this choice manifest themselves either in developing further illness or in regeneration and healing. By your mind and your expectations about life, you determine more than you think: the further course of your life.

Fundamental Solution

Take a good look into the depths: bring up your Plutonic emotions and observe them; don't be afraid of them. With your wisdom, look closely at your suppressed energies and let everything flow upwards; remove your anxieties and sadness at the surface.

Let trust, warmth, and love circulate through your total heart and body; powerfully become Master over yourself and become aware of your divinity! Enter the daylight with the riches of all your feelings!

•

Oh, ice cold snowman, please thaw out; become warmly alive (again). You can't just run away out of your warm heart; for doesn't it really beat and live in you?

---

[20] See the symbolism of Red Wine in *The Horn of Plenty*. This work has not yet been translated into English at the publication of the present book.

You've tarried enough: Come here on earth! In your shoes, on the warm soil. No longer flee. Stay close to yourself, inside yourself.

And even more, regenerate! Be reborn in an "I" that once ignored itself and now feels: life is possible again, but differently than before. A change is needed. Be full of Love for yourself, full of body warmth — instead of denying your body, throwing it away, chilling it, unfleshing it.

Time for the playful, childlike aspect in you, like a giraffe,[21] so high and joyful, with its tongue in the leafy tree crowns: you now descend again into your earthly soul. Happily come back to yourself, being with yourself, delighted to be who you are as an "I" on earth. Acknowledge your body of flesh and blood, that childlike playfulness, the power of your bones, and the flexibility of eternal youth in you.

Say yes to love, to yourself, to your body, to life, to your "I" within this beautiful life.

Everything depends on *how* you look at life; on how you look at yourself; on whether you make the unconditional CHOICE of a thankful existence — strong in self-love.

Nothing can be promised. You don't need to feel guilty about anything, and certainly not about this illness. But do come wholeheartedly INTO yourself; give yourself every chance.

See also: page 5 to 118 of the present book; if applicable, see also: Colorectal Cancer. See also, in *The Key to Self-Liberation:* Cancer, in General; the chapter about the psychological correspondence of the intestines, and especially the part of the intestine where the disease originated.

Colorectal Cancer
cancer of the large intestine
bowel cancer, colon cancer,
rectum cancer

Fundamental Origin

While slowly pondering, the human being sucks a tobacco pipe; he dreams of promising perspectives, full of expectation.

But does he live with both feet on the ground? Does he decide not to close his eyes to reality — including his acceptance of its less pretty sides? Then, this will be shown to him later on, by life itself.

"Speak up, express yourself," says life, "Dreaming, standing still, thinking, indulging in illusions, won't get you any further. What is *true* reality, what are *real* values?"

Have you become thought, dream, intoxication . . . instead of being your *true* "I," in reality? Your "I" of flesh and blood, no longer fleeing away into distant spheres with dreams and thoughts?

Are you building a false palace? Do you attach importance to money or other values, which in fact are not values?

Life urgently calls you back into yourself: so that you would learn to appreciate your real treasures and talents — that which is highest and most noble in you — and let go of the lower.

This doesn't mean that you are a "bad" person, but it does mean that *you lose yourself* in values that are not true values.

This is the psychological image with which this illness can be compared. As if you are asked to come with both feet into the here and now, sober-mindedly, and to not dwell in intoxication or false joy. To no longer hide behind something or someone but to fully manifest yourself. To express yourself from out of your FEEL-

---

[21] The special symbolism of the giraffe is explained in depth in the book *If Animals Could Talk. . . .* This work has not yet been translated into English at the publication of the present book.

INGS, your true "I," your Heart. Also to say what is *really* going on in your mind — to not bottle anything up inside you.

While grinding your teeth, so to speak, in order to not have to show your feelings and thoughts or to be able to keep them in check, you hold tight under your arm your precious possession, whatever this may be (for instance, material possessions, a title, a diploma, appearances, children, friends, a partner, a performance, an emotional secret, etc.). Do you attach importance to material values? Do you want to keep so much with you? Are you afraid of having to give up something of yourself — literally and/or figuratively, materially and/or emotionally — or are you angry at having to do so?

As if you are mad at the world, as if you fear being short of something or are afraid that others would take something away from you.

This tenacity, this distrust, this hiding, won't get you any further. You feel wronged as though someone else would be the cause of your "suffering."

Fundamental Solution

Know, then, that nothing is a coincidence — that in your life you attract everything on the basis of your convictions, be it unconsciously.[22]

Therefore, with an eye for reality, you have every reason to open your hands in a joyful and trusting way to that which life wants to offer you — without desiring or wanting to have or possess something or someone.

Clear up the dirt in the now. And certainly don't be "pissed of" about things which after all you have attracted yourself. Don't think about the lower. You are being asked to perform a clean sweep inside yourself.

Dare to look at the unsavory, the negative, which you may have kept with you so far, like a non-seeing person.

Go in search of **true** values; cease to cherish illusions, false romance, dreams (or paradises of lies). Let go of **everything** that doesn't belong within the realm of the **true** Values inside you, the Values that reign in the kingdom of Life.

Let go while loving yourself, while communicating openly with other good-hearted people, without pushing your underlying feelings aside. Lovingly **give** to yourself, to others.

Let go; let go also of things from the past that annoyed you.

Let go in peace, love, tranquility, and understanding, so that you can build your true paradise on earth, on the basis of your own, genuinely beautiful, essential values. Be happy and thankful about this.

See also, in *The Key to Self-Liberation*: Cancer, in General; Large Intestine, in General.

HEART PALPITATIONS: EXTRASYSTOLES
Your heart skips a beat

Fundamental Origin and Solution

Your legs, *tired* and walked on until they are bowed, as it were, dead-tired. You finally don't know anymore how far you have gone already, *for how long you have been persevering in this direction* (literally or figuratively), but one thing is definite: it has been going on for a long time! But you keep on going on and on and on, so that your legs might take on

---

[22] Read more about this on page 5 to 118 of this book.

an O shape. You probably think *it all HAS TO BE that way,* just like the long distance runner or jogger who is totally convinced that this or that distance *must* be covered: *that it is supposed to be that way,* or for the sake of fitness; in the meantime one doesn't realize that one causes oneself to grow older and shrink instead of becoming healthier, but one is convinced that it *is* okay, no matter how much effort it costs!

Life itself doesn't ask for this. Why such insistent, fixed ideas? Why still live according to "oppressive laws" without questioning them? *Use YOUR INDIVIDUALITY, your highly unique thinking Ability, in order to place it all in question . . . and to see where you constantly FORCE, EXHAUST, push yourself, where you do things that are hard for you, where you absolutely keep it up and don't even question: "Is this LIFE; is this really good for me?" Then stand still . . . and think about this. See how you have forced yourself to keep on walking in a tense way for too long, have acted or thought strenuously in this or that direction, in this or that hard way.* Now take away those blinders.

Stop "following," doing what's "supposed to be done," what others, or society, norms, and rules tell you to do "because it's good for you." FOLLOW YOUR HIGHLY UNIQUE PATH in a loving, but truly creative way. After all you are not a monkey, not an imitator, not an idiot who runs in circles or does this or that every night because "someone" says that's how it's supposed to be . . . that's how it has to be . . . as if YOU are not allowed to exist as YOU! As if life asks you for strong efforts!

Time to change the rudder: you live from your inner Feeling, from your heart. It's okay for you to work and make efforts, build up thoughts, but as long as they don't hurt you, as long as they are not "pushed on you" by doctrines, habits, social norms or whatever. You do take responsibility for your existence, but you now begin to live from out of your creative "I"-thinking and your supervising brain!

Stop walking on in this way. Reconsider everything. Look at *where* you just do and follow what the rules and others and society have told you to do: realize then that LIFE doesn't ask that from you. *IN-DEPTH UNDERSTANDING is being asked; possibly seeing through certain indoctrinations which make you give importance to things of no importance.* Go back to the source inside yourself and ask yourself what's GOOD for YOU personally.

An *example:* don't live automatically or think that sport is healthy because everyone says so. Know why you need this or that food product and why your body enjoys it, no matter if it's chocolate or pears. Know that nothing is unhealthy if the signal comes from out of your deepest self, from your soul-center upwards, and tells you to take this or that. But at the same time understand the cause of your liking this or that food product, and work at it.[23] A human being is HEALTHY when he JOYFULLY experiences his own nature and does what he feels he has to do, from out of his deepest self — not because it "has to be that way" or because that's "the way it's done."

BE . . . BECOME who you *really* are! Also regarding the exterior: don't allow yourself to be fooled into believing that only skinny muscles are healthy, and fat would inevitably be unhealthy, that you have to be slim at all costs, and being

---

[23] Please note that there are important conditions attached to this. See the chapter "Food and Health" in this book.

heavy would automatically be bad or un-healthy. FEEL what is good and healthy for you, and also see through the cult of looks and appearances: true beauty lies in the extension of truth, not in someone who creates a body made to manipulate with power, emptied inside and filling himself with things and/or people from the outside.

No longer ACHIEVE on any level, but just be yourself: live according to the truth, from your heart, in goodness, and *SEE THROUGH* things, look for *the ES-SENCE,* for *the CONTENT* of life, no longer FORCING yourself in order to GET, *to want TO HAVE* this or that. *Let go! Arrive at the vibration of BEING in-stead of HAVING!* And this "having" doesn't necessarily have anything to do with material things (although this is also possible), but it can be about *"wanting to have a certain situation" that is not there (yet)* . . . and you WANT this to come to be. *LET GO! Don't force anything; and trust. Experience the joy of your "Being."*

Stop making it so hard for yourself, stop also FILLING yourself with the things you think to be IMPORTANT but which in fact in the view of Life itself are of no im-portance. Listen to that gentle but reso-lute voice of your inner heart and follow only that path. Don't live on the SUR-FACE, on the outside of your being, but live and act from out of your deepest source, according to what you feel deep inside. *It's necessary to look THROUGH things,* to realize thoroughly that every-thing has a reason.

DON'T JUST KEEP ON WALKING ON AND ON without coming to the realiza-tion of the fact that there lies something MUCH deeper under the surface and false layers — search for that information of truth. This can be done by no longer thoughtlessly doing things the way you used to, by no longer keeping on going in a direction you used to think you were

supposed to go in. Now listen to your in-ner ear. WHAT does your heart really want? *What* does life ask?

No longer make yourself so tense. No longer fill yourself with things, but EXPE-RIENCE YOURSELF in your own full-ness; enjoy your being. Don't just be oc-cupied with your work, or with just what you do or achieve, but *connect yourself with your INNER CORE OF FEELING, with your heart; then FEEL how it calls for a "stop," NOT KEEPING ON RUNNING the way you are at the moment . . . in thoughts and meditations or in deeds.*

Return to your deepest source, turn deeply inward, be good and gentle with yourself. Stop "filling" yourself, and now fulfill yourself completely with the love that will flow through your total being. *For a while stop living, thinking, working, organizing at the Surface . . . and listen to the deep, wonderful voice of what you Feel inside, of your heart.* No longer tire yourself; don't exhaust yourself in thoughts or in deeds.

No longer keep on walking on that way — but in a very loving way reflect on yourself and dig deeply for the ES-SENCE of life, of yourself. You no longer live out of your *Head,* out of *Obligation,* but out of your total being, out of what you feel in your middle, out of your warm navel region, where life begins. You live out of what you feel inside, you live out of love, and you fill yourself with new life-energy — resting a bit — no longer run-ning on the way you used to.

Stay very close to yourself, to this heart of yours; *no longer concentrate on the outside of things, people, matter; nor lin-ger by outer factors and material details.* But *essentially* turn toward that which will nourish you, and in such a way that in-stead of shrinking, wasting away and de-generating, you will constantly regener-ate yourself: now you lovingly FEED your body.

A warm glow, an energy full of love, flows through your entire body. Your cells continuously renew themselves. You warm and feed yourself. You no longer run past yourself.

The life energy comes from within . . . and you feel that now, and you now open yourself up to it. *You stop for a moment of reflection about yourself and don't rush yourself with your head, with indoctrinations, duties, norms, thoughts . . . . No, you now continuously STAY close to your heart; your thoughts / mind / spirit are not separate from your body. Your heart-energy now feeds every fiber of your body: doing good, giving rest; warming and giving health.* You feel yourself growing in this inner power and rest. Steadily, you do your tasks in life, no longer taking leave of your "I," your heart, your body. You are *One* — in the alliance with yourself, according to heart, soul, and body.

You no longer skip yourself, the Essence of yourself . . . you no longer run along till you fall down exhausted. You live according to your inner being, and every chilly distancing from your body, your heart, from what you feel inside, has disappeared.

You don't live in the tower of your thinking, but very intensely and connected with mother earth. *A delightful coziness in matter; very close to your inner "I," and never again will work, thoughts, details, the superficialities, etc., get the upper hand. You are gentle and full of love, one in unification with yourself, according to heart and soul.* You take the time to reflect on yourself. Whenever you do something, no matter what, you no longer "separate" yourself from yourself, you no longer just run on. You don't do ANYTHING — with your head, your thoughts, or just out of habit — without your HEART and your BODY being in-

volved with it! *Only in this way will you FEEL when you are running away from Life, or whether you stay present in your Heart, your body, your total being while doing or thinking. You no longer skip the essence of yourself, of life . . . and your heart doesn't skip a beat anymore either.*

YOU ARE . . . NOW. You no longer RUN just anywhere in the desire to obtain something or get somewhere — whether it has to do with insisting on finishing a work or reaching a finish line or running the kilometers "someone" tells you is healthy. You no longer want to get "somewhere," no longer want to "endure," from your head, from your programmed *fixed ideas,* from your acquired convictions, because this destroys life. *You no longer insist on getting something "done," fixated in your head in a hard way: you let go and you arrive now at the essence of yourself, in love and mildness.* You now question everything and arrive at your true Heart: you learn to feel what life asks of YOU. Nothing is a "must". . . . Except "listening to this essential feeling of life," listening to your heart, to what your heart tells you is good for you.

Don't dwell on unimportant external factors or details. Live according to the essence . . . and Be who you ARE; remain always present with this BEING and don't "force" yourself into anything. Goodness and love count — not achieving, shining or responding to false ideals. Live and experience yourself in love, from the Core of your "I." Don't demand things from yourself . . . but LIVE out of the joy of your total, unified essence. Come into deeply felt contact with your heart, your body, your content of treasures. *You no longer force anything; you no longer want to obtain anything; therefore, you no longer get angry, in impatience or nervousness. You live out of goodness, in thankfulness for your being, looking at the Content, the Essence of things, people, life.*

ATRIAL FIBRILLATION OR FLUTTER

goes together with a very irregular heartbeat

Fundamental Origin

Painfully wounded, as if someone has given you a thrust in the stomach; but it's you yourself who first stabbed yourself in the stomach, as it were. You harshly hurt yourself and attract painful situations as a result. Born with the conviction that you have to defend yourself, are vulnerable, and have to perform things with a rough red hand. Piled-up aggression, blind anger sometimes; a pugnacious spirit and a kind of death urge. The hands — and the heart — ask to be allowed to give in love, and to thankfully receive from life. But you grab hold of things or people, you believe that you have to defend yourself, being convinced that existence is a calvary: one person's death and another person's salvation, but not for long. There's that misery again, that combativeness, the fire in you which is stirred up by your convictions that life is a battleground ruled by the power of the strongest and that you always need to defend yourself — attack is the best defense — because somehow you want to see "blood": this represents an unconscious urge to arrive at more "life." You won't solve this by standing in life in a desirous, angry, aggressive, combative way — by living in struggle or by losing yourself in hot-blooded emotions and burning desires (covetousness, sex without love, wanting to get others to do certain things, etc.). Everything you need is IN you. Don't expect it from the outside. Desire and anger go together.

Anger because you don't obtain what you want to "have," is lethal.

Fundamental Solution

Now let go of things and people, and turn inward. Chop off that dead, grabbing, black-charred hand; *solve the primordial, entrenched problem deep inside yourself. Don't blame it on others nor attribute it to events from the past:* these were only a consequence of your outlook. So change this attitude toward life; live according to a *loving, gentle,* understanding mentality. As a result, life circumstances will change also. *Take yourself into life in a warm-hearted, loving way. Come more into yourself, into your body of "flesh and blood."* Thankfulness for your being, for everything that IS now; *enter into your BE-ING.* Don't grab for more and more in endless repetition: that's how you take yourself out of life. Break with an old pattern in which you fooled yourself into believing that you would always be short of something, that you would have to fight, grab, seize, possess, and desire for your existence, that you would need to position yourself in life with as much aggressive powers as possible: this is the path of death. So, unhook yourself!

Chin up! *Acknowledge the divine human being in yourself — the royal messenger who you are. Proclaim life in all its colors. How marvelous this is.*

*Let go, **give**, **live**, in love and peace.* Why continue to suffer, fight, sorrow, die? *This isn't necessary.* Live according to the conviction that Life asks for nothing better than that the human being would go along with it on its frequency, that he would choose an eternal and everlasting Covenant.[24] The desirous, aggressive, grasping, clenching, clinging hand has now been chopped off — figuratively speaking.

---

[24] More about this in the book *New Days*. This work has not yet been translated into English at the publication of the present book.

No more heated, angry or pugnacious thoughts. Come home to yourself in a "mild-hearted" manner. *And the heart pumps calmly, but powerfully, into the direction of that one road that is called "Life."* You no longer desire. You "are" happy about who you are. No more harshness. The sword has been put down. Gratitude flows through your heart.

MALIGNANT MELANOMA

a type of cancer that develops from the cells that produce the skin-darkening pigment called melanin

Fundamental Origin

You wipe dirt from the path with a straw witch-broom that is *far too feeble.* You keep sweeping incessantly; but seemingly the longer you brush, the fuller and wider the broom becomes and the more dirt accumulates under it. Instead of going away, the specks of dust and dirt multiply. So it seems to be a magical broomstick that asks for a *turnabout,* also in you.

Because there is insufficient POWER — *healthy, strong-willed Life Force* — behind the weaponry (*the immune system*), it fades and weakens whereas the instrument is actually intended to be used to GET RID of all filth. This only makes matters worse. The more the sweeping is done in such a feeble way, the more the body experiences itself as impotent, limp, feeble when it comes to realizing oneself and defending oneself against "the evil" — in this case against the intruder called cancer.

A multiplication of the negative — of *that which the Human Being should remove inside and outside himself, with full commitment, force, and his whole heart.* Why this faintness!!? Why give the chance to the dirty dust, that which is lifeless, to multiply? By your limp attitude in life, your lack of genuine drive, of active assertiveness, your energetically pale manner, you stimulate, as it were, this expansion or rise of the negative. In this way indeed your immunity breaks down.[25]

The helicopter propeller blades spread out widely but *they let themselves droop in slackness.* Stagnant and not rotating, as if the helicopter *does not believe in its own ability* to turn, to get into movement. *Where is your powerful Central Core, your "I AM"-awareness?*

You carry a light, passive-pale-blue plastic bag meant to contain much in it; but it's *"empty,"* as if the human being asks himself: "So, what will I put in my shopping bag now?" Instead of moving forward vigorously, going intuitively to a shop and taking *resolutely* the things he needs. No. Loitering, hesitating, *"I don't know."* It doesn't seem like you intend to "fill" the bag in a meaningful way. You seem to experience life, to step into it, in a faint and feeble way. You are *not really CONSCIOUSLY present, in yourself and near to yourself;* you just let it all happen. STOP! STAND UP!

No longer allow yourself to *"be lived."* You are not a demihuman, are you? You are a POWERFUL, divine human being who fulfills himself, isn't it? Or do you think you have to "fill" yourself as if you were empty? You don't mean it! Filling yourself with things, people, drink, sex, ostentation, TV, constantly doing this or that on the surface of life?!

---

[25] Please read in the present book the chapters about *Immunity.* Also, the chapters about *HIV-AIDS* are not only written for AIDS patients, but for all people whose immune system is weakened.

Fundamental Solution

Get up with might and main! Bang your fist on the table: "Heck, I AM, I LIVE, and I FEEL my powers. From now on I will employ THE FORCE that is in me. I am not a limp, empty schmuck who has no say over himself anymore! *I grab myself by the collar; with full self-awareness and high resolve I take My Life in hand; I arrive at TRULY BEING AS "I,"* yes, at truly ACTING. Self-realization from out of the BELIEF in YOURSELF: that is your salvation.

You don't let yourself be thrown off your balance; you stand up for yourself. NEVER again will you allow yourself to droop, that's your firm decision. Enough! Over and done! You break definitively with a certain vision on yourself, on life. *Hercules* is your example: he defeated the five-headed monster. You defeat the voice in you that fooled yourself into believing that you were incapable of anything, worthless, that your forces could not or cannot surface. With the power of a GIANT you go onward in Life.

Dauntless, intensely CONCENTRATED in every muscle fiber of your body. Consciously present on Earth as "I"!

Please read also the text *Cancer, in general* in *The Key to Self-Liberation.*

FAT, FATTY TISSUE

Fat, by itself, is Good and Healthy, Soft and Beautiful. In the present decades however, Western society is oriented toward the notion that fat is ugly and unhealthy.[26] Here we talk about "Fat" in the "healthy, fleshy human being" as well as the thin layer of fat in the "healthy, lean human being." The following text does not apply to chubbiness accompanied by health problems.

Many people — and especially women — are slaves of this destructive conviction, and they violate themselves just to make "fat" melt away in a manner that is too radical, by forcing themselves (e.g., extremely strict diets, liposuction, etc.). This is unnatural and unhealthy.

"Live according to Life!" is the essential answer here;[27] **then you will see what is your specific, natural, healthy fat content. This is different for each individual.**

Feelings and potential possibilities for Creativity — which are extensive but don't have to be transformed right away into action and realization — are Energies. These energies may be solidified into Fat. *Fat should not disappear so long as it is necessary for the human being (at the level of physical and psycho-emotional health).*

Fat symbolizes Energy, Potentiality, Self-Cherishing, and Gentleness. Without a physical collection base for the enormous energies that are present in the nature of certain people, these people would become ill or insane. (It's completely normal that many people who begin following an unnaturally strict "diet" may be confronted by one or another ailment.)

The balance between Energy (feelings, potential creativity, etc.) and Body, between spirit and matter, constantly needs to be maintained in a natural way.

Therefore, you are fine the way you are at any moment in your existence, so long as you don't mold yourself into an artifi-

---

[26] On the other hand, there are societies other than the present Western one who wrongly worship fat.

[27] Read about this on page 5 to 118 of this book.

cial straitjacket, so long as you "live on the wavelength of Life"! Read more about this on page 5 to 118 of this book.

If you don't feel fine, then follow only your inner Authority, which gives you the body that is ideal for you at this moment. Fat, by itself, is not ugly or bad — on the condition that you live "according to Life." Don't fight against this, but be in solidarity with your beautiful, soft, warm, powerful, downy body, which retains its muscles and layers of fat where they are needed for your health. No longer look at fat through the eyes of a society which only lives superficially and doesn't know true love. A society in which the woman and the man are being proclaimed as instinctive suction-powers instead of as Human Beings who incarnate full love that *gives*.

Listen to your heart, to your body: don't listen to superficial counselors who can't get to the bottom of things because they, themselves, are swallowed up by these destructive convictions.

A body shape reflects the individual nature of a human being.
*Certain "fat places" make it clear to you why it has formed just **there**: and it is good. It doesn't have to disappear.*

Stand up for who you really are; don't hide behind a false "suction-mask" of a "reducing diet, slim-down massage," etc. And *if* the fat at some point should disappear either spontaneously or following a consciously chosen, healthy, balanced weight-loss process, then your deepest Self will also know that this is good. And should it spontaneously come back at a certain moment, then this has its reasons. However, read the paragraph below entitled "The above text does not apply to . . . ."

Don't live according to the standards of the outer world, but from out of your deepest Nature, from your true Being: then you will see where it is good to have fat on your body. If at a certain moment energies "liquefy" and the exteriorization of your content breaks through, then also some fat disappears: you "change" in a way. Then this loss of fat or weight is good.

Learn not to "lie" to yourself by, for instance, "losing weight" whereas actually it's your nature to be round. Only then will you meet a friend, a partner, who loves YOUR rounded nature of being and not a sham image.

If a friend only "takes" you because (and as long as) you meet the requirements of this or that thin-shape-without-fat, then there's no question of genuine love for your Genuine Being. Let go; no longer throw pearls before swine. Open yourself in love to those friends who wish to truthfully share that golden treasure in you (the heart, the fat, the love, the gentleness . . .).

And discover the rounded beauty — on the condition that it is shaped from out of the heart, of course. Because well-rounded people may also draw in, attract, seduce by their flesh-and-fat-shapes. This, then, is not the path that leads to Life in health.

The above text does not apply to:

- People who suffer from a malfunction of certain glands (for instance, thyroid, adrenals, hypophysis, pancreas . . .). In these cases, the basic problem is not the fat in itself but the underlying illness or the malfunction of a certain organ. Then read the relevant texts: ailments of the thyroid gland, in general, and the psychosomatic solutions; ailments of the adrenal glands, in general, and the fundamental solutions; etc.
- People who have an urge to eat without being really hungry, or without putting into practice what this phenomenon asks them to do.
- People who do not succeed to live "according to Life." (See page 5 to 118.)

FEELING A STRONG NEED FOR EATING SUGAR OR SWEETS

In itself, sugar certainly isn't unhealthy.[28]

Sugar is fuel that immediately warms you and can give you a pleasant feeling if you are open to it. Because you long for love, warmth, sweetness, you quickly reach for "sweet' products.

By itself, it is not an addiction to like sweet products such as sugar, but it is a natural need for what you, with your individual disposition, so much long for: sweetness, gentleness in life.

Enjoy sugar products, then, and don't refuse sugar in a condemning way. But it is true that your fondness for sugar is a signal from yourself, which makes clear to you: be nice to yourself; fill yourself with the warm fuel of yourself, with love.

If eating sugar products is accompanied by anxious, compulsive behavior instead of calm enjoyment of something sweet, then this indicates that you experience yourself too much as an emptiness, as a coldness, that you are not really present in your "body," that you deny — don't really allow — the sensuality in yourself, the pleasantly sweet sensorial aspect, the enjoyment of earthly things, of your sensuous longings!

You determine your being, with dark thoughts; perhaps you attach much importance to the exterior, to your "facade" and allow yourself to be misled by social demands and norms concerning the cult of looks and appearances. Nothing of all this is of importance. Love yourself; develop emotional warmth, which is the true fuel for your body, dare to be yourself the way you are, in joy.

Don't force a harsh, tough, strict "diet" on yourself (except, of course, when this is necessary for medical reasons), but enjoy sweetness. If you feel attracted to this, you need to take sweet products on the condition that you no longer leave yourself out in the cold, considering yourself a zero.

Sugar is being completely assimilated and digested only if you are firmly and Consciously aware of your Worth, if you are nice to yourself, and if you direct your creative energies outward. Be productive in whatever area, and don't allow yourself to listlessly run empty.

Don't grasp, don't hold on to things or people. Direct your radiating forces, your love, *outward!* Unfold yourself; don't retain your forces and your possibilities.

Don't be sad; don't put yourself in a subordinate, dependent position. Be proud of yourself; get a hold on yourself, not on others!

Become aware of your rich Content, of your inner Fuel, the forces of love and trust in yourself, which constantly nourish your total body, so that you no longer *have to* eat sugar, but still may.

Don't be hard and strict on yourself; feel full of self-confidence, and no longer *let* yourself "be lived." Allow feelings to flow freely, and resolutely determine your course of life.

Life is joy: discover that warm, feeling core inside you; yield to love for yourself so that you no longer feel "lonely." Only when you are convinced that you are

---

[28] However, diabetics will first have to work on the psychological origins of their disease before the pancreas can function normally again and little by little the intake of sugar can rise again (under the supervision of a competent doctor who acts in accordance with the present knowledge of medical science, who understands psychosomatics, who is capable of judging whether medicine or insulin need to be administered and in what dose, and whether at a certain point it is possible to progressively diminish the dosage when the patient's living self gives signals to do so).

"worthy" of love, happiness, and warmth, will you attract joyful circumstances.

Bring about changes regarding your expectations of life, so that you create happiness yourself. Enjoy the earthly, and don't push it away.

It's allowed to eat sugar products on the condition that you are nice to yourself now, because the pancreas will function optimally only under impulses of self-love. The longing may remain, and the satisfying of this longing also may remain, but the "imperative need" will disappear in proportion to the growth in yourself of emotional warmth.[29]

TYPE 2 DIABETES

**in adults, elderly persons;
formerly called 'mature onset diabetes'
or 'old-age diabetes'**

Fundamental Origin

Something in you seems to say "No!" in a harsh way, bunched up with anger, your neck strained, your head pulled in between hunched shoulders; maybe with a clenched fist. As if you don't want to see your own face anymore; it seems like you don't really want to be in touch with yourself anymore. A cross refusal to continue living in this way. As if you doom yourself and your life. Forces conglomerate in powerlessness — in refusal.

Yes, it's about a refusal to be gentle with yourself, to give yourself the warmth and the love that you need so much. You are so hard on yourself, so angry, so unwilling to allow yourself to be who you are, with the utmost love! As a consequence, you expect this from others — but this is impossible. First *give* it to yourself. First, say "yes" to yourself. Only then can you enter into a harmonious loving relationship with the other person. Stop this sharp self-destruction. You may find it very difficult to get out of the existing situation. You nail yourself to the ground, to the cross, as it were, refusing to take a single step farther. You can't go on anymore; you don't want to anymore.

You push yourself away, in gray realms — instead of discovering yourself with joy and coming out with who you are. As if you don't love yourself at all, don't love your body or a part of it, don't love your becoming "older." (You can be eternally young! In the name of goodness, don't see "beauty" according to the indoctrinated norms of society. Know that, for instance, children aged 5-10 years often look very "old." Know that true beauty radiates from within; it radiates outward through the body. *This* beauty is everlasting and entails eternal youth![30])

It's as if you put demands on life — sometimes with immoderate desire — and as a result are furious because life doesn't give you this or that, or because others don't want to meet certain expectations of yours. Know then that every desire — everything you absolutely "want to obtain" from others or from life — is a symbol of that which you lack inside yourself. You want to "have" something, to "get" someone to do something, because you're not content about who you ARE. As a consequence you want to "fill"

---

[29] Attention: there are important conditions attached to this. See the chapters "Living in Harmony with Life" (p. 21), and "Food and Health" (p. 74). Also read more about this in *The Symbolism of Food — The Horn of Plenty*. This work has not yet been translated into English at the publication of the present book.

[30] Read more about this on page 5 to 118 of this book, in the book *New Days,* and in the psychological symbolism of the star named "Duo" in the book *On Earth as in The Heavens.* The two last mentioned works have not yet been translated into English at the publication of the present book.

your life; you want to compensate for your feelings of dissatisfaction, possibly by expecting things from others or by feeding anger against others inwardly. But deep down yourself you know that in this way you are erring and you can't stand the sight of your own face anymore, so to speak; you no longer want to look "into your own eyes." There's an utter resistance to who you *really* are.

Fury rages because of your immense powerlessness to arrive at self-love; there's sometimes self-hatred or self-rejection, there's impatience, anger, sometimes a frenzy. You'd like to fight, roar, rant and rave, because you don't want to see yourself anymore, but you tensely restrain yourself; you remain silent and hide yourself behind your high coat collar or under your hat. In the end, you possibly don't want anything more to do with the others; you don't want any contact, neither with yourself nor with others. You obstinately close yourself off.

At the same time, there may be the pull of a kind of suction force, asking attention or love from the others, wanting to draw them toward you, wanting to glue yourself affectively to the other person, with desire. It's up to you now to recognize that desire, suction, having expectations from others, have nothing to do with life and love but with death and illness.

The "female" aspect of you is too passive and, at the same time, too prone to grab — giving too little love in an active way, to yourself in the first place; the "male" aspect is too hard, too dominant, too demanding, too condemnatory toward yourself. Both aspects complement each other well as regards negative orientation. They now need to be definitively reversed within your personality structure.

Fundamental Solution

Arrive at higher awareness; from out of your heart, in thankfulness, direct yourself to that which is Higher in you. That's where happiness lives, that's where contentment lives! You can no longer grab; instead, *give* attention to yourself, to others, with an open heart.

Don't coop yourself up; no longer harshly run yourself down in a destructive, self-negating way.

Are you angry with "the other person," with life — because you think that they are ill-intentioned, that they don't give you what you need? You are the only one who can give you what you need: the noble recognition of your entire self, the destruction of the angry, ungrateful "animal" within yourself.

So, come closer to your heart and climb to those noble heights in yourself. That's where you will find peace; that's where there's room for TENDERNESS, AFFECTION, LOVE, and a THANKFUL EXPERIENCE of yourself, of life, of good-hearted people around you.

Anchor yourself deeply into your own essence — and manifest yourself open-facedly. No longer hide angrily, but open your sight to the beautiful things that life wants to reveal to you!

Say yes to yourself, to Life as it offers itself; then, from out of this atmosphere of gratitude, you can direct your Life yourself toward a beautiful future.

Know that, as soon as you allow demands, desires, anger, harshness, self-destruction, and suction within yourself, you actually banish yourself from life.

Come *very* close to your heart; open yourself to the most GENTLE atmospheres within yourself. Allow primordial, caressing, "skin-soft" female energies within yourself — warm, giving love — to stream in.

Do not grab, let go; do not angrily clench yourself together but unfold yourself. Open up, no longer resist thawing. It's not the others, it's not life that don't give you what you would want to have; you alone are the one who, unconsciously or consciously, attracts everything, but really everything, on your life path.

Therefore, it's in your best interest to consciously make something beautiful out of your life. Don't ask anything from others; expect everything from yourself. In this loving restoration of contact with yourself, you will also find peace with everything and everyone in your surroundings.

Relaxation. Loving recognition. Accepting yourself with open arms. Inner peace. Letting go.

"Surrender" to that which your Living Self-Essence expects of you. You now OPEN yourself up. You surrender to the Love toward Life, toward yourself at the level of your "soul" and "body" — in gratitude for your "being," in eternal youth, in true beauty from out of the Heart: YOU!

Human Being Loves Human Being

THE "MALE" AND "FEMALE" ASPECTS IN EVERY HUMAN BEING

Smashing Up Old Idées Fixes

Hetero, homo, hermaphrodite? Asexual? Transsexuality, Transgender?

These terms do not indicate illnesses but dispositions. Every human being is unique, not equal to anyone else.

Let's start with those people who experience themselves to be "**transsexual**" or "**transgender**." Some among them feel the need to let themselves be **operated** upon in order to transform their bodies from one sex to another, others don't at all. I fully sympathize with people who were born in what is commonly called a "woman's body" but have the feeling of being a "man," and who therefore con-

sider gender reassignment surgery in order to transition into what is commonly called a "man's body." Or vice versa. But, out of love for these people, I ask them, **don't mutilate yourselves**. Whether you opt for surgery or not — you, as free human beings — please take some time to quietly reflect on the text below.

•

In the following chapter I address myself to **all** human beings.

JUST LET US CONSIDER THINGS THROUGH THE EYES OF THE LIFE'S HEART.
Who will determine "what" "a woman" is and "what" "she" should "look like"?
Who determines "what" "a man" is and "what" "a man" should "look like"?

Everything goes well as long as the Human Being *recognizes* in himself the life-aspects that one generally associates with *"the feminine"* as well as those aspects that could be called *"masculine"* — I will continue to use these terms — *bringing both into harmonious union within his own "I."*

The so-called feminine aspects, in a positive sense: the intuitive, sensitive moon aspect, the receptiveness, the capacities of releasing, giving birth from out of oneself, turning deeply inward, taking care of others, etc.

The so-called masculine aspects, in a positive sense: powerfully manifesting oneself, like a rock rising above the water, proud as a peacock illuminated by the sun, like an architect who vigorously pushes his way through the jungle in order to construct a world, thrusting ahead, etc.

Both aspects, left and right, what is commonly called feminine and masculine.[31] This can be considered on a primitive, instinctive level, there were the human-animal instinct still fully dominates.

OR one transforms these primal aspects into a higher level where love and being-aware prevail — behold the Human Being who has become conscious and has left behind him the stadium of the human animal.

The meaning of Life is that humanity evolves and — in so doing — brings Life itself further along, until even physical death, as the ultimate disease, will be overcome. Because the physical body (every cell, every gene, . . .) immediately reacts to convictions and thoughts that exist in the spirit.

Energy and matter are interchangeable (cf. Einstein); but what is much more important is that the Human Being — when he becomes aware of it — is capable of directing the body and its "energy" with his Spirit that has become Conscious. Toward happiness and health when steered by Love, toward illness and perishing when steered by ignorance, power, or evil.

To this day, there hasn't been much "conscious" steering or directing; in his *unconscious state* of "being," the human being has lived according to customs and convictions such as: "There's no escape from dying; so, in order to ensure the survival of 'the species,' an 'offspring' has to be created."

Up to now, this has led mostly to the "Tarzan-and-Jane-Syndrome" (at least in Western society; things went differently elsewhere): the weak little female calls for help and "draws" the so-called tough, imposing male toward her. The urges to entice and to capture meet in the sexual game.

In our world, men and women behave according to this old instinctive pattern and bear "their" children. Sexually provocative postures, maneuvers of seduction, the corresponding attire in the world of fashion all belong to this "animal-human-race."

This is an observation, not a condemnation; every human being is free to live in this way or not.

As a human being, it is possible that you notice certain signals (feelings, occurrences, experiences) at a certain moment in your life — signals that make you see things completely differently; while living with Love in your heart, you may, for instance, not (or no longer) feel like having sex and may feel the need to step out of the above-mentioned customs and conducts.

You feel yourself being born as a New Human Being,[32] not in order to die, but to live. This goes very far and can seem implausible to you as a reader, but maybe this won't be the case anymore at a certain point in the future.

Keep in mind, nothing is obliged! Everything is evolution; a further step is made when the time is ripe for it. Nothing must be forced. Every human being does well to follow his personal "signals."

●

Regarding the true, newborn Human Being, such as LIFE itself intends him to be within the evolutionary process:

1) He experiences both aspects — "the feminine" and "the masculine" — *inside*

---

[31] See also in *The Key to Self-Liberation,* the texts about the two hemispheres of the brain, the left and right sides of the body.

[32] Read more about this subject in *New Days* (not yet published in English at the time of the publication of the present book).

of himself; in this evolution, he grows toward the COMPLETE HUMAN BE-ING.

2) He no longer feels the need to concentrate on "the exterior": "I want others to find me beautiful and attractive." He *loves himself* and he *gives,* he is able to love ANOTHER HUMAN BEING.

3) **So, whether one is born into a body that is commonly called male or female does not play a role anymore. One has become A HUMAN BEING.**

4) Inwardly, certain men or women will identify with the feminine rather than with the masculine aspect (or vice versa); it would be a good thing if they learned the lesson to still **further develop in them the other aspect as well**.

5) Sexuality is not the same as Love. So far, one has expressed sex either in an animal manner or in a humane, loving manner, but **in itself, sex is not to be equated with "Love."** Certain people do not like it, others do. Nothing is "obliged."

6) **Whether it's about what one calls a man and a woman — or two men, or two women, or two people of androgyne nature — who love each other, this is of no importance whatsoever to Life. Love can be passed on FROM ONE HUMAN BEING TO AN-OTHER HUMAN BEING, in the greatest tenderness, while truly *giving* — not attracting or drawing in. Love is Life.**
Grabbing and drawing in (like the pull of a suction force) lead to death. In fact, the terms hetero, homo,

transsexual, transgender would better not be used altogether.
HUMAN BEING LOVES HUMAN BE-ING, WHETHER OR NOT ACCOMPA-NIED WITH PHYSICAL EXPERI-ENCES. Being aware, however, that sex-without-love lies on the paving stones of the path of death. True Love *gives* Life! Sex is not the main thing; it is a possibility, not a must. Most likely it is even a transitional stage in the history of Humankind.[33]

7) And what if the person whom one calls a woman would have three breasts . . . or no breasts at all? What if she would have a penis, testicles, and a hairy chest? And what if the person whom one calls a man would have breasts and no penis?
This isn't the point at all, is it?
And who determines what kind of clothes one should wear?
Here, the **division**, the schizoid situation in humankind comes to light: the disease to be solved that once arose and developed in humanity as a whole. One has "labeled" black-and-white what should be called "a man" and what should be called "a woman." This is, in other words, **the PIGEONHOLE MENTALITY** in which one should belong to 1 category (as determined by oneself and/or society).

8) **True physical beauty can only be perceived by the human being who "forms" and experiences his body FROM OUT OF THE HEART**, love. This has nothing to do with the so-called "beauty norms" that prevail in society — empty, dead, fake, false "beauty," herd syndrome, fashion slave, aesthetics of death. And then one can hear other people say, people who do not live truly: "Oh, you are so

[33] Read more about this subject in the text "Transformation" within the chapter "Sex, Hormones, Sexuality."

beautiful!" Whereas you are actually on the path of false beauty and death. In this way you can never become happy. For it's about an image one wants to reach for oneself (desire); one disappears in it. One loses oneself in "the other image," in "the other one" — amorous self-loss like Narcissus, not living. One wants to catch the eye, be seen; one would do anything in order to "possess." From this angle, plastic surgery molds an even deathlier image. It ISN'T beautiful. One strays away far from oneself while sometimes manipulating others.

Search your way back to your TRUE "I," FEEL YOUR HEART, love yourself the way you are, body and soul. This authentic beauty is healthy, makes you and other people happy. Being labeled "MAN" or "WOMAN" is of NO IMPORTANCE to life and love, dear HUMAN BEING!

9) Let go of the aesthetics of death. Striving after an **"outward model," with perfectionism** — but disconnected from the heart and "seen" **through the eyes of death** — is fatal. The aesthetics of death: in order to please, to seduce, to be "the most beautiful" (allegedly). **This image of "APPEARANCE"** makes one sick and unhappy because **it IS NOT beautiful** — the human being is just not aware of this. Being cut off from one's truth essence, one doesn't know anymore what is really beautiful. In this perfectionist atmosphere of outward appearance one desires attention, but this "desire to possess," *to attract the eye,* etc., lies on the path of gradually dying away.

It is no wonder that, despite much surgery, one never becomes satisfied or happy, and that some people even end up taking their own lives. It is only in one's own natural BEING — when the body has been shaped from within, in love that *gives* — that one is beautiful, with each remaining faithful to his unique nature. Love and goodness, the ONLY TRUE, honest beauty: the way one IS by nature. No narcissism but generosity of heart, whatever one "looks like."

Fundamental Solution?

If all human beings would feel themselves to be HUMAN BEINGS — living from out of the loving heart, uniting in them both aspects: that which one now calls feminine and masculine — THEN THERE IS NO QUESTION ANYMORE OF BEING FIXATED ON THE "EXTERIOR," on the physical form in itself. Then, also, operations are superfluous (in the meaning of plastic surgery or gender operations).

Healing of the Human Being: the heart content and the form, the exterior, correspond to each other. *The Healthy human being does not bother himself about "what one should look like" in order to be called either a man or a women.* Let alone that the healthy human being, who has become aware and is full of love, would behave, dress or speak with "mannerism."

People who experience themselves as transsexual or transgender do well to realize also that they are okay as a man-woman or as a woman-man, whatever they look like. And that, as long as a man born in what one now calls a male body who says of himself, "I am a homosexual," or, "Inwardly, I am actually a woman but I live in a man's body and I am transgender,"[34] wants to use specific gestures in his behavior or even considers undergoing sex reassignment sur-

---

[34] The same goes for "the woman" who feels herself to be "a man," or other possible variations.

gery to get a woman's body, then he hasn't understood that this is not what LIFE is about.

This show, **the cult of external appearance, disconnected from the Two-oneness that lives in every Human Being**, man-woman, is aimed at attracting attention, seducing, drawing others toward one, capturing — the illness called "dying." Sexual instincts, grabbing.

Being full of love, loving oneself: that is what it's about. Whether you experience yourself as homo, hetero, transgender . . . Love for yourself. Love for someone else (whatever the disposition of the other person may be).

LIVE! In Love

IT DOESN'T MATTER AT ALL HOW YOU DRESS, HOW YOU BEHAVE, . . . **Recognize your full humanity, the man and the woman *in* yourself**. Don't act the tough guy like Tarzan, don't play the feeble or cool person like a whore — this goes as well for those who call themselves homosexual as for heterosexuals or transgenders. Do not want to catch the eye but love yourself. Do not want to be the "mask model," walking artificially, inauthentic, disrupted, just playing a "role," far removed from being naturally yourself. Put a stop to the "false light," to putting up a show. Simply be . . . yourself.

BECOME A HUMAN BEING. LIVE FROM OUT OF YOUR HEART — BODY AND SOUL.
LOVE YOURSELF THE WAY YOU WERE BORN.
FEEL THE PRIMAL FEMALE FORCE inside yourself.
FEEL THE PRIMAL FEMININE SOFTNESS inside yourself.
FEEL THE PRIMAL MALE FORCE inside yourself.
FEEL THE PRIMAL MASCULINE SOFTNESS inside yourself.

ONE kind of HUMAN BEING:
the divine human being who is full of love;
and *don't bring your body into question.*

Feeling and experiencing your man-woman-oneness from the inside,
the exterior plays no role anymore . . .
unless you prefer to remain a "human animal."

Who says that a woman doesn't have a penis?
Who says that a man doesn't have breasts?
Who DESIGNATES what, and in what way? All has been "pigeonholed" within a society that is built more on "wanting to possess" than on "being" in happiness. *But the beloved true Life doesn't know any pigeonholes or labels; therefore, it doesn't know operations that consolidate the labeling pattern either.*
Letting oneself be operated on (for instance, sex reassignment surgery or liposuction) is a form of self-destruction — mutilating yourself and not loving yourself unconditionally.

One is stuck in *old "patterns" :* this is how a man MUST be, feel, and behave; and, this is how a woman MUST feel inwardly, look like, and behave.

The newly born Human Being does not talk of "sex" but of "love." He or she is not interested in how he or she looks like, in whether he or she gets attention from people of this or that "sex."

If hetero women want to show themselves as limp, weak, smiling Janes or as cool temptresses, they don't respect Life. If those who feel themselves to be homosexual or transgender / transsexual also want to manifest the same gestures and mannerisms — thinking also that they have to wear plunging necklines and shake their bottoms, for instance — then the hetero woman (Jane) as well as the man who wants to imitate this behavior as a homo or a transgender / transsexual (wanting to be "like that" comes from within) are both on the path of perversity and are not truly Living.

Conversely, the same goes for the so-called lesbian "woman" — or the "woman" who calls herself transgender / transsexual — who, for instance, who wants to show herself to herself and others as a bearded, tough, well-muscled person.

Come to life — integrate the TRULY feminine and the GENUINELY masculine into yourself, whether you were born in what one now calls a man's body or a woman's body.

Transform yourself inwardly into **the two-oneness-divine-human-being that you are, who is potentially present in every human being**. No longer identify yourself with either the one or the other "sex," because then you deny **your magnificence as a Human Being full of Love**.

Moreover, true beauty can only be seen in a human being who lives in love and can give from out of his heart. What body form? That's totally unimportant. Operations are superfluous.

Love, love, **true self-love . . . and, possibly, sharing love with one another; two complete human beings love their physical appearances as outward expressions of "I AM." They no longer feel the need (the desire) to "look" like this or like that, nor to be called "a beautiful woman" or "a beautiful man." Oh yes: a marvelous human being full of love!**

●

The way you have looked at it is very understandable. However, it is time now to treat yourself as a Worthy Human Being, to see things differently. You are full of love and no longer linger over this issue.

You no longer want to incline toward just one side. *You are the MAN-WOMAN-human-being whose body form carries a wealth of love. Whether it be with our without penis, with or without breasts, with or without growth of hair in this or that region of the body — THAT is of no importance whatsoever to the TRUE human being, to LIFE itself.*

Be thankful for who you are on the plane of content and form, whatever they may be like. Happy human being! *No self-mutilation but self-love, while experiencing your fullness. The New Human Being. Overcome the condition of being split by putting an end to the "pigeonhole mentality."*

Do you experience yourself to be transgender or transsexual?

If, as a transgender / transsexual human being, you really want to "catch the eye" or "attract attention," then it is recommendable that you read the above text.

Now come to that powerful, loving oneness core of Man-Woman within yourself; recognize your full value, wanting no longer to "attract notice."

Love yourself as "a Human Being," then the need disappears to be "seen" or approved by others.

Know that **the only living norm of beauty that exists is** the human being who lives FROM OUT OF LOVE, from out of GIVING, in a loving way (not from out of "instincts," seduction, grabbing, wanting to be found sexually attractive).

THAT IS THE TRULY BEAUTIFUL HUMAN BEING. The human being who transforms primeval instincts into consciousness energies that are full of love. He loves himself; he is dynamically creative for the good of the human being and humanity.

You are not one of the herd, not "a physical appearance"; you are a FULLNESS in being unique, by uniting man and woman in your "BEING."

Bid farewell to the stupid cult of "outward appearance." Be happy about who you ARE as HUMAN BEING.

Go to the core, the essence of yourself; there you can experience "who" you really are: a HUMAN BEING who carries in him the masculine as well as the feminine aspect.

You develop mastery over your creative powers; you construct your life, as a human being.

You give yourself loving attention instead of expecting this from others.

Dear Human Being,
I love you the way you are,
in the goodness of
your Being.

MEMORANDUM